ZEN SEATS

CHAIR YOGA MASTERY

FOR VIBRANT SENIORS

HENRY I. GREAT

"Zen Seats: Chair Yoga Mastery for Vibrant Seniors"

Copyright © 2024 by Henry I. Great

All rights reserved. No part of this publication may be reproduced, distributed, or transmitted in any form or by any means, including photocopying, recording, or other electronic or mechanical methods, without the prior written permission of the publisher, except in the case of brief quotations embodied in critical reviews and certain other noncommercial uses permitted by copyright law.

"Zen Seats: Chair Yoga Mastery for Vibrant Seniors"

TABLE OF CONTENTS

CHAPTER ONE 5
  1.1 INTRODUCTION 5
    1.2 Welcome to the World of Chair Yoga 6
    1.3 Understanding the Benefits of Chair Yoga for Seniors 9
    1.4 Setting Intentions for Your Chair Yoga Journey. 12

CHAPTER TWO 15
  2.1 GETTING STARTED WITH CHAIR YOGA 15
    2.2 Exploring the Basics: Breath, Alignment, and Mindfulness 18
    2.3 Selecting the Right Chair and Setting Up Your Space 21
    2.4 Warm-up Exercises to Prepare Your Body and Mind 24

CHAPTER THREE 28
  3.1 CHAIR YOGA POSES FOR STRENGTH AND FLEXIBILITY 28
    3.2 Gentle Stretches to Improve Flexibility and Joint Mobility 38
    3.3 Building Strength and Stability through Seated Asanas 42
    3.4 Enhancing Balance and Coordination with Chair Yoga Flows 46

CHAPTER FOUR 51
  4.1 Relaxation and Stress Relief Techniques 51
    4.2 Guided Relaxation and Visualization Practices .. 59
    4.3 Breathing Exercises for Calmness and Clarity 63

"Zen Seats: Chair Yoga Mastery for Vibrant Seniors"

4.4 Using Props and Modifications for Comfort and Support 68

CHAPTER FIVE 73

5.1 CHAIR YOGA FOR EVERYDAY LIFE 73

5.2 Integrating Chair Yoga into Daily Routines: A Comprehensive Guide 77

5.3 Integrating Chair Yoga into Daily Routines: A Comprehensive Guide 80

5.4 Mindful Movement for Improved Focus and Energy 84

CHAPTER SIX 89

6.1 CHAIR YOGA FOR SPECIFIC HEALTH CONCERNS .. 89

6.2 Managing Arthritis and Joint Pain with Chair Yoga 93

6.3 Alleviating Back Pain and Improving Spinal Health with Chair Yoga 97

6.4 Nurturing Mind, Body, and Spirit: The Holistic Approach to Well-being 101

CHAPTER SEVEN 105

7.1 CULTIVATING SELF-COMPASSION AND ACCEPTANCE THROUGH CHAIR YOGA 105

7.2 Connecting with Others through Chair Yoga Communities and Classes 109

7.3 Embracing Aging Gracefully with Chair Yoga Wisdom 113

CHAPTER EIGHT 117

CONCLUSION 117

"Zen Seats: Chair Yoga Mastery for Vibrant Seniors"

CHAPTER ONE

1.1 INTRODUCTION

Welcome to the World of Chair Yoga

Dear Reader,

Congratulations on taking the first step towards a journey of vibrant health, renewed vitality, and inner tranquility. In this transformative guide, "Zen Seats: Chair Yoga Mastery for Vibrant Seniors," we embark together on an exploration of the ancient art of yoga adapted specifically for individuals over 55 years old.

Chair yoga offers a gateway to wellness that is accessible to everyone, regardless of age or physical ability. Whether you're new to yoga or a seasoned practitioner, this book is your comprehensive companion to harnessing the power of yoga from the comfort of your chair.

As we age, it's natural for our bodies to undergo changes, and with those changes often come new challenges. Chair yoga provides a gentle yet powerful approach to maintaining and improving physical health, mental clarity, and emotional well-being. Through a combination of gentle movements, breath work, and mindfulness practices, chair yoga empowers you to cultivate strength, flexibility, and resilience in both body and mind.

In these pages, you'll discover not only the physical benefits of chair yoga but also its profound impact on your overall quality of life. From enhancing flexibility and mobility to reducing stress and promoting relaxation, chair yoga offers a holistic approach to aging gracefully and joyfully.

"Zen Seats: Chair Yoga Mastery for Vibrant Seniors"

Throughout this journey, I encourage you to approach your practice with an open heart and a curious mind. Embrace each moment with a spirit of self-compassion and non-judgment, allowing yourself to explore and discover the unique gifts that chair yoga has to offer.

Whether you're seeking relief from chronic pain, longing for a deeper sense of connection with yourself and others, or simply curious to explore new possibilities, "Zen Seats" is here to guide you every step of the way.

So, take a seat, breathe deeply, and let the transformation begin.

With gratitude and warmth,

[Henry I. Great]

1.2 Welcome to the World of Chair Yoga

Chair yoga is a gentle yet powerful practice that opens the door to the transformative benefits of yoga for individuals of all ages and physical abilities, particularly seniors over 55 years old. In this welcoming introduction, we'll explore what chair yoga is, its origins, and why it's such a valuable practice for promoting holistic well-being.

What is Chair Yoga?

Chair yoga is a modified form of yoga that adapts traditional yoga poses and practices to be performed while seated or using a chair for support. It incorporates gentle stretches, breathing techniques, meditation, and mindfulness exercises to promote physical health, mental clarity, and emotional balance.

"Zen Seats: Chair Yoga Mastery for Vibrant Seniors"

Origins of Chair Yoga

The roots of chair yoga can be traced back to the ancient traditions of yoga, which originated in India thousands of years ago. Traditionally, yoga was practiced on the ground, with practitioners sitting, standing, or lying on yoga mats or rugs. However, as yoga has evolved and adapted to meet the needs of diverse populations, including those with mobility issues or physical limitations, chair yoga emerged as a way to make yoga accessible to everyone.

Why Chair Yoga?

Chair yoga offers numerous benefits that make it an ideal practice for seniors over 55:

1. **Accessibility**: Chair yoga eliminates the need to get up and down from the floor, making it accessible to individuals with mobility issues, joint stiffness, or balance concerns.

2. **Safety**: By providing support and stability, the chair reduces the risk of falls or injury during yoga practice, making it a safe option for seniors.

3. **Gentleness**: Chair yoga poses are gentle and low-impact, making them suitable for older adults who may have arthritis, osteoporosis, or other chronic conditions.

4. **Flexibility**: Chair yoga can improve flexibility, range of motion, and joint mobility, helping seniors maintain their independence and quality of life.

"Zen Seats: Chair Yoga Mastery for Vibrant Seniors"

5. **Stress Reduction**: Chair yoga incorporates relaxation techniques, such as deep breathing and guided meditation, which can help seniors reduce stress, anxiety, and depression.

6. **Community**: Chair yoga classes provide an opportunity for seniors to connect with others, build friendships, and share experiences in a supportive and inclusive environment.

What to Expect

In "Zen Seats: Chair Yoga Mastery for Vibrant Seniors," you'll find a comprehensive guide to chair yoga designed specifically for individuals over 55. Whether you're new to yoga or have been practicing for years, this book will provide you with everything you need to begin or deepen your chair yoga practice.

Throughout the book, you'll explore a variety of chair yoga poses, breathing exercises, relaxation techniques, and mindfulness practices. Each chapter will offer step-by-step instructions, modifications, and tips to help you customize your practice to suit your unique needs and abilities.

So, if you're ready to embark on a journey of self-discovery, healing, and transformation, take a seat, open your heart, and let the magic of chair yoga unfold.

Welcome to the world of chair yoga—a world of possibility, empowerment, and profound well-being.

1.3 Understanding the Benefits of Chair Yoga for Seniors

As we age, maintaining and promoting overall well-being becomes increasingly important. Chair yoga emerges as a powerful and accessible tool for seniors over 55, offering a myriad of physical, mental, and emotional benefits. Let's delve into a comprehensive exploration of why chair yoga is a valuable practice for the senior community.

Physical Benefits

1. **Improved Flexibility and Range of Motion:**
   - Chair yoga involves gentle stretches and movements that enhance flexibility, helping seniors maintain or regain range of motion in joints and muscles.

2. **Enhanced Strength and Stability:**
   - Seated poses and modified standing poses in chair yoga contribute to building strength in the core, legs, and arms, promoting better balance and stability.

3. **Joint Health and Pain Management:**
   - Gentle movements in chair yoga promote joint health and can be effective in managing chronic pain associated with conditions like arthritis or stiffness.

4. **Better Posture and Spinal Health:**
   - Focus on alignment and mindful movements in chair yoga helps seniors develop better

posture and supports spinal health, reducing the risk of back issues.

Mental and Emotional Benefits

1. **Stress Reduction and Relaxation:**
    - Incorporating deep breathing exercises and relaxation techniques, chair yoga provides a sanctuary for seniors to release stress and tension, fostering a sense of calm and relaxation.

2. **Enhanced Cognitive Function:**
    - Mindful movements and breathwork stimulate the mind, promoting cognitive function and mental clarity, which is particularly beneficial for seniors looking to maintain cognitive health.

3. **Mood Regulation:**
    - Regular chair yoga practice has been associated with improved mood and reduced symptoms of anxiety and depression, contributing to emotional well-being.

4. **Mind-Body Connection:**
    - Chair yoga encourages seniors to connect with their bodies, fostering a deeper awareness of sensations, emotions, and the present moment, promoting mindfulness.

"Zen Seats: Chair Yoga Mastery for Vibrant Seniors"

Accessibility and Inclusivity

1. **Adaptability for Various Abilities:**
   - Chair yoga is adaptable to different physical abilities, making it accessible for seniors with varying levels of mobility, flexibility, or strength.

2. **Reduced Risk of Injury:**
   - The use of a chair provides support, reducing the risk of falls or strains, making chair yoga a safe option for seniors concerned about balance or stability.

Social and Community Benefits

1. **Connection and Community:**
   - Participating in chair yoga classes offers seniors an opportunity to connect with like-minded individuals, fostering a sense of community and social engagement.

2. **Shared Experience:**
   - Sharing the chair yoga journey with others provides a supportive environment where seniors can exchange experiences, challenges, and triumphs, creating a sense of camaraderie.

Understanding these multifaceted benefits underscores the importance of chair yoga as a holistic practice tailored to the unique needs of seniors. "Zen Seats: Chair Yoga Mastery for Vibrant Seniors" will guide you through harnessing these benefits, empowering you on your journey towards a healthier, more fulfilling life.

1.4 Setting Intentions for Your Chair Yoga Journey

Embarking on a chair yoga journey is not merely about physical movements; it's a holistic endeavor encompassing mind, body, and spirit. Setting intentions at the outset of your chair yoga practice can infuse your journey with purpose, mindfulness, and direction. Here's how to set powerful intentions for your chair yoga journey:

1. Cultivate Awareness

Begin by bringing awareness to your current state—physically, mentally, and emotionally. Reflect on your reasons for starting a chair yoga practice. Are you seeking relief from physical discomfort? Longing for mental clarity or emotional balance? By acknowledging your starting point, you lay the foundation for intentional growth and transformation.

2. Clarify Your Goals

Identify specific goals you wish to achieve through your chair yoga practice. These goals could be physical, such as improving flexibility or managing pain, or they could be more holistic, such as cultivating inner peace or enhancing overall well-being. Clarifying your goals helps you align your intentions with your desired outcomes, providing clarity and focus as you embark on your journey.

"Zen Seats: Chair Yoga Mastery for Vibrant Seniors"

3. Set Positive Affirmations

Craft affirmations that reflect your intentions and aspirations for your chair yoga practice. These affirmations should be positive, empowering statements that resonate deeply with you. For example, "I am grateful for my body's strength and flexibility" or "I cultivate peace and serenity with each breath I take." Repeat these affirmations regularly during your practice to reinforce your intentions and cultivate a positive mindset.

4. Embrace Mindfulness

Integrate mindfulness into your chair yoga practice by paying attention to the present moment with openness and curiosity. Mindfulness allows you to deepen your connection with your body, breath, and sensations, fostering a sense of presence and inner peace. Set the intention to approach each practice with mindful awareness, savoring the richness of each movement and breath.

5. Practice Self-Compassion

Extend kindness and compassion to yourself as you embark on your chair yoga journey. Recognize that progress takes time and that each step forward, no matter how small, is worthy of celebration. Set the intention to treat yourself with gentleness and understanding, embracing both your strengths and your limitations with love and acceptance.

6. Stay Open to Possibility

Maintain an open heart and an open mind as you engage in your chair yoga practice. Stay curious and receptive to the lessons and insights that arise along the way. Set the intention to remain flexible and adaptable, embracing the unexpected twists and turns of your journey with grace and resilience.

7. Cultivate Gratitude

Finally, cultivate an attitude of gratitude for the opportunity to embark on this chair yoga journey. Reflect on the blessings in your life, both big and small, and set the intention to approach your practice with a heart full of gratitude. Gratitude opens the door to abundance and joy, enriching your chair yoga experience with a sense of wonder and appreciation.

By setting intentions for your chair yoga journey, you empower yourself to cultivate growth, healing, and transformation on all levels. May your intentions guide you along the path to greater well-being, vitality, and inner peace.

CHAPTER TWO

2.1 GETTING STARTED WITH CHAIR YOGA

Embarking on your chair yoga journey is an empowering step towards enhancing your well-being and vitality. Whether you're new to yoga or a seasoned practitioner, starting with chair yoga offers a gentle and accessible entry point to the practice. Here's how to get started on your chair yoga journey:

1. Establish Your Space

Create a dedicated space for your chair yoga practice—a quiet, clutter-free area where you can focus and move comfortably. Choose a sturdy chair without wheels, preferably with a straight back and no armrests. Place your chair on a non-slip surface, such as a yoga mat or carpet, to ensure stability during your practice.

2. Dress Comfortably

Wear loose, comfortable clothing that allows for ease of movement. Opt for breathable fabrics that won't restrict your range of motion. Remove any jewelry or accessories that may interfere with your practice. The goal is to feel relaxed and unrestricted as you move through your chair yoga poses.

3. Warm-Up

Begin your practice with a gentle warm-up to prepare your body and mind for movement. Start by sitting comfortably in your chair with your feet flat on the floor. Take a few deep breaths, inhaling through your nose and exhaling through your mouth. Gently roll your shoulders back and forth, loosen your neck with gentle neck rolls, and rotate your wrists and ankles to release tension.

4. Mindful Breathing

Focus on your breath throughout your chair yoga practice. Practice mindful breathing by inhaling deeply through your nose, feeling your belly expand, and exhaling slowly through your mouth, feeling your belly contract. Use your breath to anchor your awareness in the present moment and cultivate a sense of calm and relaxation.

5. Explore Basic Poses

Begin with simple chair yoga poses that gently stretch and mobilize your body. Experiment with seated twists, side stretches, forward folds, and gentle backbends to increase flexibility and improve circulation. Modify poses as needed to suit your comfort level and physical ability. Remember to listen to your body and honor its cues.

6. Focus on Alignment

Pay attention to proper alignment in each pose to prevent strain and injury. Sit tall with your spine lengthened, shoulders relaxed, and feet grounded firmly on the floor. Engage your core muscles to support your posture and maintain stability. Align your knees over your ankles and your hips over your knees to maintain balance and integrity in your poses.

7. Embrace Modifications

Don't hesitate to use props and modifications to support your practice. You can use cushions, blankets, or yoga blocks to provide additional comfort and stability in certain poses. Modify poses by adjusting the range of motion or intensity to suit your individual needs and limitations. Remember that chair yoga is adaptable to all bodies and abilities.

8. Conclude with Relaxation

Finish your chair yoga practice with a period of relaxation and reflection. Sit quietly in your chair, close your eyes, and take several deep breaths. Release any tension or stress held in your body, allowing yourself to fully unwind and let go. Offer gratitude to yourself for showing up on the mat and dedicating time to your well-being.

9. Stay Consistent

Commit to a regular chair yoga practice to experience the full benefits over time. Aim to practice at least a few times per week, gradually increasing the duration and intensity of your sessions as you progress. Consistency is key to reaping the rewards of chair yoga and cultivating a deeper connection with yourself.

By following these steps, you'll lay a solid foundation for your chair yoga practice and embark on a journey of self-discovery, healing, and transformation. Embrace each moment on the mat with openness, curiosity, and compassion, knowing that you're nurturing your body, mind, and spirit with every breath.

"Zen Seats: Chair Yoga Mastery for Vibrant Seniors"

2.2 Exploring the Basics: Breath, Alignment, and Mindfulness

In the realm of chair yoga, the fundamentals of breath, alignment, and mindfulness serve as the cornerstone of a transformative practice. By delving into these essential elements, you'll unlock the full potential of your chair yoga journey, cultivating awareness, presence, and inner harmony. Let's explore each of these basics in depth:

1. Breath

The breath is the life force that animates our bodies and connects us to the present moment. In chair yoga, conscious breathing serves as a powerful tool for calming the mind, energizing the body, and deepening our practice. Here's how to harness the power of breath in your chair yoga practice:

- **Deep Belly Breathing:** Begin by sitting comfortably in your chair with your spine tall and shoulders relaxed. Place one hand on your belly and the other on your chest. Inhale deeply through your nose, allowing your belly to expand as you fill your lungs with air. Exhale slowly through your mouth, feeling your belly gently contract. Repeat this deep belly breathing pattern several times, syncing your breath with your movements.

- **Ujjayi Breath:** Experiment with ujjayi breath, also known as "ocean breath," to create a soothing and rhythmic sound that calms the mind and regulates the nervous system. Inhale deeply through your nose, slightly constricting the back of your throat to create a whisper-like sound. Exhale audibly through your nose, maintaining the gentle constriction. Allow the sound of your breath to guide you deeper into relaxation and presence.

2. Alignment

Proper alignment is essential for optimizing the benefits of chair yoga poses, ensuring safety, stability, and efficiency of movement. By paying attention to alignment cues, you'll cultivate greater body awareness and prevent strain or injury. Here are some key alignment principles to keep in mind:

- **Spinal Alignment:** Sit tall with your spine lengthened and your shoulders stacked directly over your hips. Engage your core muscles to support your posture and prevent slumping or rounding of the spine.

- **Joint Alignment:** Align your knees directly over your ankles and your hips over your knees to maintain stability and balance in seated poses. Avoid hyperextension or locking of the joints, keeping a gentle micro-bend in your knees and elbows.

- **Shoulder Alignment:** Roll your shoulders back and down, away from your ears, to open up the chest and create space in the upper body. Draw your shoulder blades together slightly to broaden across the collarbones and release tension in the shoulders.

3. Mindfulness

Mindfulness is the practice of bringing non-judgmental awareness to the present moment, cultivating a sense of clarity, acceptance, and presence. In chair yoga, mindfulness allows us to deepen our connection to ourselves and the world around us, fostering inner peace and well-being.

"Zen Seats: Chair Yoga Mastery for Vibrant Seniors"

Here's how to integrate mindfulness into your chair yoga practice:

- **Body Scan:** Take a few moments at the beginning of your practice to scan your body from head to toe, noticing any areas of tension or discomfort. Bring gentle awareness to these sensations without judgment, allowing yourself to release and relax with each breath.

- **Sensory Awareness:** Notice the sensations of your breath as it flows in and out of your body, the feeling of your feet grounded on the floor, and the subtle movements of your muscles as you transition between poses. Cultivate a sense of curiosity and openness to the present moment experience.

- **Anchor Point:** Choose an anchor point, such as the sensation of your breath or the feeling of your feet on the ground, to bring your attention back to whenever you notice your mind wandering. Use this anchor point as a grounding tool to center yourself in the present moment and cultivate mindfulness throughout your practice.

By exploring the basics of breath, alignment, and mindfulness in your chair yoga practice, you'll lay a solid foundation for growth, healing, and transformation. Embrace each moment with openness, curiosity, and compassion, knowing that you're nurturing your body, mind, and spirit with every breath.

2.3 Selecting the Right Chair and Setting Up Your Space

Creating a conducive environment for your chair yoga practice is essential to ensure comfort, safety, and enjoyment. By selecting the right chair and setting up your space mindfully, you'll optimize your ability to engage fully in your practice and reap its myriad benefits. Let's explore everything you need to know about selecting the right chair and setting up your space for chair yoga:

1. Choosing the Right Chair

Selecting a suitable chair is the foundation of your chair yoga practice. Look for a chair that meets the following criteria:

- **Sturdy and Stable:** Choose a chair that is stable and secure, with four sturdy legs and a solid frame. Avoid chairs with wheels or swivel mechanisms, as they may compromise stability during your practice.

- **Comfortable Seating:** Opt for a chair with a comfortable, cushioned seat that provides adequate support without being too soft or too firm. The seat should be wide enough to accommodate your hips and thighs comfortably.

- **Straight Back:** Look for a chair with a straight backrest that supports proper spinal alignment. Avoid chairs with overly reclined or slouched backs, as they may encourage poor posture during your practice.

- **Armrests (Optional):** While not essential, chairs with armrests can provide additional support and stability, especially for individuals with mobility issues or balance concerns. If you choose a chair with armrests, make sure they are at a comfortable height and do not restrict your movement.

2. Setting Up Your Space

Creating a dedicated space for your chair yoga practice enhances focus, tranquility, and mindfulness. Follow these steps to set up your space mindfully:

- **Clear the Area:** Choose a quiet, clutter-free area with enough space to move comfortably around your chair. Remove any obstacles or distractions that may disrupt your practice, creating a peaceful and inviting environment.

- **Non-Slip Surface:** Place your chair on a non-slip surface, such as a yoga mat, carpet, or rubber floor, to ensure stability and safety during your practice. Avoid practicing on slippery or uneven surfaces that may increase the risk of slips or falls.

- **Natural Light and Ventilation:** Whenever possible, practice in a space with ample natural light and ventilation to create a bright, airy atmosphere conducive to relaxation and rejuvenation. Open windows or doors to let in fresh air and natural sunlight, uplifting your mood and energy levels.

- **Personalize Your Space:** Add personal touches to your practice space to create a warm and inviting ambiance. Consider incorporating elements such as plants, candles, or inspirational quotes to inspire and uplift your spirit during your practice.

- **Tech-Free Zone:** Create a tech-free zone by turning off electronic devices or placing them out of sight during your practice. Minimizing distractions from phones, computers, or TVs allows you to fully immerse yourself in the present moment and connect with yourself on a deeper level.

3. Accessibility Considerations

If you have mobility challenges or specific accessibility needs, consider the following adjustments to make your chair yoga practice more comfortable and inclusive:

- **Chair Height:** Adjust the height of your chair to ensure that your feet can rest flat on the floor with your knees bent at a comfortable angle. Use cushions or blocks to raise or lower the seat height as needed to achieve proper alignment.

- **Chair Positioning:** Position your chair near a wall or sturdy surface for added support and stability during standing poses or balance exercises. Use nearby furniture or props for additional assistance and safety as required.

- **Modifications and Props:** Explore modifications and props, such as cushions, blankets, or straps, to adapt poses and movements to your individual needs and abilities. Modify poses to accommodate any physical limitations or discomfort, focusing on comfort and safety above all else.

By selecting the right chair and setting up your space mindfully, you create an environment that supports and enhances your chair yoga practice. Approach each practice with an open heart and a sense of curiosity, knowing that you're nurturing your body, mind, and spirit with every breath.

"Zen Seats: Chair Yoga Mastery for Vibrant Seniors"

2.4 Warm-up Exercises to Prepare Your Body and Mind

A thoughtful warm-up routine is essential for priming your body and mind for a fulfilling chair yoga practice. By incorporating gentle movements, stretches, and breathing exercises, you'll increase circulation, flexibility, and mental focus, setting the stage for a deeper and more enriching experience. Here are some warm-up exercises to help you prepare your body and mind for chair yoga:

1. Seated Neck Rolls

- Sit comfortably in your chair with your spine tall and your shoulders relaxed.
- Inhale deeply, lengthening through the crown of your head.
- On an exhale, gently lower your chin towards your chest, feeling a stretch along the back of your neck.
- Inhale as you roll your right ear towards your right shoulder, stretching the left side of your neck.
- Exhale as you roll your chin back towards your chest.
- Repeat on the opposite side, rolling your left ear towards your left shoulder.
- Continue alternating sides, moving slowly and mindfully with your breath.

2. Shoulder Circles

- Sit tall with your feet flat on the floor and your hands resting on your thighs.

- Inhale deeply as you lift your shoulders towards your ears, scrunching them up.
- Exhale as you roll your shoulders back and down, drawing your shoulder blades together.
- Continue to roll your shoulders in a circular motion, moving them up, back, down, and forward.
- Focus on creating smooth, fluid movements, releasing tension and stress with each rotation.
- Repeat for several rounds, then reverse the direction of the circles.

3. Seated Cat-Cow Stretch

- Sit comfortably in your chair with your feet flat on the floor and your hands resting on your thighs.
- Inhale deeply as you arch your spine, lifting your chest and drawing your shoulder blades together (Cow Pose).
- Exhale as you round your spine, tucking your chin towards your chest and drawing your belly button towards your spine (Cat Pose).
- Flow between Cat and Cow Pose with your breath, moving slowly and with awareness.
- Focus on mobilizing your spine and synchronizing movement with breath, creating space and flexibility in your back.

4. Seated Side Stretches

- Sit tall with your feet flat on the floor and your hands resting on your thighs.

"Zen Seats: Chair Yoga Mastery for Vibrant Seniors"

- Inhale deeply as you reach your right arm overhead, lengthening through your fingertips.
- Exhale as you gently lean to the left, feeling a stretch along the right side of your torso.
- Hold the stretch for a few breaths, then inhale to return to center.
- Repeat on the opposite side, reaching your left arm overhead and leaning to the right.
- Continue to alternate sides, moving with your breath and exploring the full range of motion in your side body.

5. Seated Forward Fold

- Sit tall with your feet flat on the floor and your hands resting on your thighs.
- Inhale deeply as you lengthen through your spine, lifting your chest.
- Exhale as you hinge forward at your hips, keeping your back straight and leading with your chest.
- Place your hands on your shins, ankles, or the floor, depending on your flexibility.
- Hold the forward fold for a few breaths, feeling a gentle stretch along the back of your legs and spine.
- Inhale to slowly rise back to an upright position, stacking your vertebrae one by one.
- Repeat thc forward fold several times, moving with your breath and gradually deepening the stretch.

6. Deep Breathing Exercises

- Sit comfortably with your feet flat on the floor and your hands resting on your thighs.

- Close your eyes and take a few deep breaths, inhaling through your nose and exhaling through your mouth.

- Place one hand on your belly and the other on your chest.

- Inhale deeply, feeling your belly expand as you fill your lungs with air.

- Exhale slowly and completely, feeling your belly gently contract as you release the breath.

- Continue to breathe deeply and rhythmically, focusing on the sensation of your breath moving in and out of your body.

- Use your breath as an anchor to center yourself in the present moment, quieting the mind and preparing for your chair yoga practice.

By incorporating these warm-up exercises into your chair yoga routine, you'll create a nurturing and supportive foundation for your practice. Approach each movement with mindfulness and intention, listening to your body's needs and honoring its wisdom. With each breath and stretch, you'll cultivate a deeper connection to yourself and pave the way for a fulfilling and transformative chair yoga experience.

"Zen Seats: Chair Yoga Mastery for Vibrant Seniors"

CHAPTER THREE

3.1 CHAIR YOGA POSES FOR STRENGTH AND FLEXIBILITY

Chair yoga offers a wide range of poses that can help seniors over 55 improve both strength and flexibility while providing support and stability. Here's a selection of chair yoga poses specifically designed to target these areas:

1. Seated Cat-Cow Stretch

- Sit comfortably on the edge of your chair with your feet flat on the floor.
- Place your hands on your knees or thighs.
- Inhale as you arch your back, lifting your chest and rolling your shoulders back (Cow Pose).
- Exhale as you round your spine, tucking your chin to your chest and drawing your belly button towards your spine (Cat Pose).
- Repeat this flowing movement, synchronizing your breath with each movement.

Benefits:

- Improves spinal flexibility.
- Releases tension in the back and neck.

How to:

1. Sit with your feet flat on the floor and hands on your knees.

"Zen Seats: Chair Yoga Mastery for Vibrant Seniors"

2. Inhale, arch your back, and lift your chest (Cow Pose).
3. Exhale, round your spine, and tuck your chin to your chest (Cat Pose).
4. Repeat the sequence for 1-2 minutes, flowing with your breath.

2. Seated Forward Fold (Paschimottanasana)

- Sit tall on your chair with your feet hip-width apart.
- Inhale to lengthen your spine.
- Exhale as you hinge at your hips and fold forward, reaching your hands towards your feet or the floor.
- Keep your back flat and your chest open, avoiding rounding your spine.
- Hold the forward fold for a few breaths, feeling a gentle stretch in your hamstrings and lower back.
- Inhale to slowly come back to an upright position.

Benefits:

- Stretches the spine, hamstrings, and lower back.
- Calms the mind and relieves stress.

How to:

1. Sit tall with your legs extended in front of you.
2. Inhale and lengthen your spine.
3. Exhale and hinge at your hips, reaching forward with your hands toward your feet.

"Zen Seats: Chair Yoga Mastery for Vibrant Seniors"

4. Keep your back straight and chest open.
5. Hold the stretch for 30 seconds to 1 minute, breathing deeply.

3. Seated Twist (Ardha Matsyendrasana)

- Sit tall on your chair with your feet flat on the floor.
- Place your left hand on the outside of your right thigh or the armrest of your chair.
- Inhale to lengthen your spine.
- Exhale as you gently twist to the right, using your left hand to deepen the stretch.
- Keep your spine long and your shoulders relaxed.
- Hold the twist for a few breaths, then return to center and repeat on the other side.

Benefits:

- Improves spinal flexibility.
- Stimulates digestion.
- Strengthens the core.

How to:

1. Sit with your spine tall and your feet flat on the floor.
2. Inhale to lengthen your spine.
3. Exhale as you twist to the right, bringing your left hand to the outside of your right knee and your right hand behind you.
4. Keep your chest open and shoulders relaxed.

5. Hold for 20-30 seconds, then switch sides.

4. Seated Side Stretch

- Sit tall on your chair with your feet flat on the floor and your hands resting on your thighs.
- Inhale to lengthen your spine.
- Exhale as you reach your right arm up and over towards the left, stretching your right side body.
- Keep both hips grounded on the chair and avoid collapsing into the stretch.
- Hold the side stretch for a few breaths, then return to center and repeat on the other side.

Benefits:

- Stretches the sides of the torso.
- Opens the chest and shoulders.

How to:

1. Sit tall with your feet flat on the floor.
2. Inhale and raise your arms overhead, clasping your hands.
3. Lean gently to one side, stretching the sides of your torso.
4. Hold for 20-30 seconds, then switch sides.

5. Seated Leg Lifts

- Sit towards the front edge of your chair with your feet flat on the floor and your hands resting on the sides of the chair for support.
- Inhale to engage your core.
- Exhale as you extend your right leg straight out in front of you, parallel to the floor.
- Hold for a few breaths, then lower your right foot back to the floor.
- Repeat with the left leg, alternating sides for several repetitions.

Benefits:

- Strengthens the quadriceps and hip flexors.
- Improves leg strength and stability.

How to:

1. Sit at the edge of your chair with your feet flat on the floor.
2. Lift one leg straight in front of you, engaging your thigh muscles.
3. Hold for a few seconds and then lower.
4. Repeat with the other leg.
5. Perform 10-15 repetitions on each leg.

6. Seated Warrior (Virabhadrasana)

- Sit towards the front edge of your chair with your feet hip-width apart and your hands resting on your thighs.
- Inhale as you lift your arms overhead, reaching towards the sky.
- Exhale as you lean slightly to the right, stretching your left side body.
- Hold for a few breaths, then return to center and repeat on the other side.

Benefits:

- Strengthens the legs and core.
- Improves balance.

How to:

1. Sit at the edge of your chair with your feet hip-width apart.
2. Extend your right leg straight behind you, toes pointing down.
3. Keep your left knee bent at a 90-degree angle.
4. Lift your arms overhead, palms facing each other.
5. Engage your core and hold for 20-30 seconds.
6. Switch sides and repeat.

"Zen Seats: Chair Yoga Mastery for Vibrant Seniors"

7. Seated Eagle Arms

- Sit tall on your chair with your feet flat on the floor.
- Inhale as you stretch your arms out to the sides.
- Exhale as you cross your right arm over your left, wrapping your forearms and bringing your palms together (or touching the backs of your hands).
- Lift your elbows slightly to deepen the stretch in your shoulders.
- Hold for a few breaths, then release and repeat on the other side.

8. Seated Warrior II (Virabhadrasana II)

- Sit tall in your chair with your feet hip-width apart and your hands resting on your thighs.
- Inhale, lengthen your spine, and lift your arms out to the sides at shoulder height.
- Exhale, turn your torso to the right, bending your right knee and keeping your left leg extended.
- Keep your gaze over your right fingertips, feeling a gentle stretch through your hips and inner thighs.
- Hold for several breaths, engaging your core and leg muscles for stability.
- Repeat on the other side, turning your torso to the left.

9. Seated Pigeon Pose (Eka Pada Rajakapotasana)

- Sit tall in your chair with your feet flat on the floor.

"Zen Seats: Chair Yoga Mastery for Vibrant Seniors"

- Cross your right ankle over your left knee, flexing your right foot to protect your knee.
- Keep your spine long and tall as you gently press your right knee towards the floor.
- Hold for several breaths, feeling a deep stretch through your right hip and outer thigh.
- Repeat on the other side, crossing your left ankle over your right knee.

10. **Seated Mountain Pose (Tadasana)**

- Sit tall in your chair with your feet flat on the floor and your hands resting on your thighs.
- Inhale, lengthen your spine, and lift the crown of your head towards the ceiling.
- Engage your core and press firmly into your feet as if you were standing on the ground.
- Hold for several breaths, feeling strong and grounded in your seated mountain pose.
- Focus on maintaining good posture and alignment throughout the pose, building strength and stability in your core and lower body.

Benefits:

- Improves posture and alignment.
- Engages core muscles.
- Stretches the spine.

"Zen Seats: Chair Yoga Mastery for Vibrant Seniors"

How to:

1. Sit comfortably with your feet flat on the floor, hip-width apart.
2. Lengthen your spine, reaching the crown of your head toward the ceiling.
3. Place your hands on your thighs or knees.
4. Engage your abdominal muscles, drawing your navel toward your spine.
5. Relax your shoulders away from your ears.
6. Hold the pose, breathing deeply for 30 seconds to 1 minute.

11. Chair Squats

Benefits:

- Strengthens the quadriceps, hamstrings, and glutes.
- Improves lower body strength.

How to:

1. Stand in front of your chair with feet hip-width apart.
2. Inhale and sit back as if sitting into the chair, keeping your knees over your ankles.
3. Exhale and return to a standing position.
4. Repeat for 10-15 repetitions.

"Zen Seats: Chair Yoga Mastery for Vibrant Seniors"

Tips for Chair Yoga Poses:

- Listen to your body and only move within a pain-free range.
- Focus on your breath, inhaling and exhaling slowly and mindfully.
- Hold each pose for an amount of time that feels comfortable for you.
- Use props like cushions or blocks for added support.

Incorporate these chair yoga poses into your routine to gradually build strength and flexibility, enjoying the benefits of a balanced and accessible practice.

NOTE: Practice these chair yoga poses regularly to build strength and flexibility while enjoying the support and stability of your chair. Remember to listen to your body and modify as needed to suit your individual needs and limitations. Enjoy the journey of exploring movement and sensation in your body, and celebrate the progress you make along the way.

"Zen Seats: Chair Yoga Mastery for Vibrant Seniors"

3.2 Gentle Stretches to Improve Flexibility and Joint Mobility

Incorporating gentle stretches into your chair yoga practice can help improve flexibility, increase range of motion, and enhance joint mobility. These stretches are designed to target key areas of the body, promoting suppleness and ease of movement. Here are some gentle stretches to explore:

1. Neck Rolls

- Sit comfortably on your chair with your spine tall and your feet flat on the floor.
- Inhale to lengthen your spine.
- Exhale as you gently lower your chin towards your chest, feeling a stretch in the back of your neck.
- Inhale to roll your right ear towards your right shoulder, stretching the left side of your neck.
- Exhale to roll your chin back towards your chest.
- Continue this circular motion, alternating sides, for several repetitions.

2. Shoulder Rolls

- Sit tall on your chair with your feet flat on the floor.
- Inhale as you lift your shoulders up towards your ears.
- Exhale as you roll your shoulders back and down, squeezing your shoulder blades together.
- Inhale to lift your shoulders up again.

"Zen Seats: Chair Yoga Mastery for Vibrant Seniors"

- Exhale as you roll your shoulders forward and down, feeling a stretch across your upper back.
- Continue this rolling motion, alternating between rolling your shoulders back and forward, for several repetitions.

3. Seated Forward Fold

- Sit towards the front edge of your chair with your feet hip-width apart and your hands resting on your thighs.
- Inhale to lengthen your spine.
- Exhale as you hinge at your hips and fold forward, reaching your hands towards your feet or the floor.
- Keep your back flat and your chest open, avoiding rounding your spine.
- Hold the forward fold for a few breaths, feeling a gentle stretch in your hamstrings and lower back.
- Inhale to slowly come back to an upright position.

4. Seated Side Stretch

- Sit tall on your chair with your feet flat on the floor and your hands resting on your thighs.
- Inhale to lengthen your spine.
- Exhale as you reach your right arm up and over towards the left, stretching your right side body.
- Keep both hips grounded on the chair and avoid collapsing into the stretch.

"Zen Seats: Chair Yoga Mastery for Vibrant Seniors"

- Hold the side stretch for a few breaths, then return to center and repeat on the other side.

5. Seated Spinal Twist

- Sit comfortably on your chair with your feet flat on the floor and your hands resting on your thighs.
- Inhale to lengthen your spine.
- Exhale as you twist your torso to the right, placing your left hand on the outside of your right thigh and your right hand on the back of the chair.
- Keep your spine tall and your shoulders relaxed.
- Hold the twist for a few breaths, then return to center and repeat on the other side.

6. Ankle Circles

- Sit tall on your chair with your feet flat on the floor.
- Lift your right foot off the floor and begin to rotate your ankle in a circular motion, first clockwise and then counterclockwise.
- Continue this circular motion for several repetitions, then switch to your left foot.
- Focus on creating smooth, fluid movements and maintaining relaxed breathing throughout the exercise.

7. Wrist Flexor Stretch

- Sit tall on your chair with your feet flat on the floor.
- Extend your right arm out in front of you with your palm facing up.

"Zen Seats: Chair Yoga Mastery for Vibrant Seniors"

- Use your left hand to gently press down on the fingers of your right hand, feeling a stretch along the underside of your forearm.

- Hold the stretch for a few breaths, then release and repeat on the other side.

- Focus on maintaining a gentle, steady pressure and avoiding any pain or discomfort.

Incorporate these gentle stretches into your chair yoga practice to promote flexibility, mobility, and overall well-being. Remember to move mindfully, paying attention to your body's sensations and limitations, and modifying as needed to suit your individual needs. Enjoy the sensation of openness and freedom in your body as you explore the transformative power of gentle stretching.

3.3 Building Strength and Stability through Seated Asanas

Seated asanas, or yoga poses, offer an effective way to build strength and stability while seated in a chair. These poses target various muscle groups and help improve overall body strength, balance, and posture. Incorporate these seated asanas into your chair yoga practice to cultivate greater strength and stability:

1. Seated Mountain Pose (Tadasana)

- Sit tall on your chair with your feet flat on the floor and your spine elongated.

- Place your hands on your thighs with your palms facing down.

- Ground down through your sit bones and lengthen up through the crown of your head.

- Engage your core muscles and press your shoulders down and away from your ears.

- Hold the pose for several breaths, focusing on maintaining a strong and stable posture.

2. Seated Warrior Pose (Virabhadrasana)

- Sit towards the front edge of your chair with your feet hip-width apart.

- Extend your right leg out to the side and bend your left knee, keeping your foot flat on the floor.

- Inhale as you reach your arms overhead, keeping them parallel to the floor.

- Exhale as you bend your right elbow and place your hand on your right thigh, reaching your left arm overhead in line with your right arm.
- Hold the pose for a few breaths, then return to the starting position and repeat on the other side.

3. Seated Chair Pose (Utkatasana)

- Sit tall on your chair with your feet flat on the floor and your knees bent at a 90-degree angle.
- Inhale as you reach your arms overhead, keeping them parallel to each other.
- Exhale as you bend your elbows and lower your hips towards the edge of the chair, as if sitting back into an imaginary chair.
- Keep your knees stacked over your ankles and your spine long.
- Hold the pose for several breaths, feeling the engagement in your quadriceps and core muscles.

4. Seated Warrior II Pose (Virabhadrasana II)

- Sit towards the front edge of your chair with your feet wide apart.
- Turn your right foot out to the side and bend your right knee, keeping your left foot facing forward.
- Inhale as you reach your arms out to the sides, parallel to the floor, with your palms facing down.
- Exhale as you gaze over your right fingertips, keeping your shoulders relaxed and your spine tall.

"Zen Seats: Chair Yoga Mastery for Vibrant Seniors"

- Hold the pose for several breaths, feeling the strength and stability in your legs and core.
- Return to the starting position and repeat on the other side.

5. Seated Tree Pose (Vrksasana)

- Sit tall on your chair with your feet flat on the floor and your hands resting on your thighs.
- Lift your right foot off the floor and place the sole of your right foot on the inside of your left thigh or calf, avoiding the knee.
- Inhale as you lengthen up through your spine.
- Exhale as you press your right foot into your left leg and engage your core muscles for stability.
- Hold the pose for several breaths, then release and repeat on the other side.

6. Seated Boat Pose (Navasana)

- Sit towards the front edge of your chair with your feet flat on the floor and your knees bent.
- Inhale as you lift your feet off the floor, bringing your shins parallel to the floor.
- Extend your arms forward, parallel to the floor, with your palms facing each other.
- Engage your core muscles and lengthen up through your spine.
- Hold the pose for several breaths, feeling the strength and stability in your core.

- Lower your feet back to the floor on an exhale.

7. Seated Twist (Ardha Matsyendrasana)

- Sit tall on your chair with your feet flat on the floor and your hands resting on your thighs.
- Inhale as you lengthen up through your spine.
- Exhale as you twist your torso to the right, placing your left hand on the outside of your right thigh and your right hand on the back of the chair.
- Keep your spine tall and your shoulders relaxed.
- Hold the twist for several breaths, feeling the engagement in your core and the stretch in your spine.
- Return to center and repeat on the other side.

Incorporate these seated asanas into your chair yoga practice to build strength, stability, and resilience in both body and mind. Remember to move mindfully and honor your body's limitations, modifying as needed to suit your individual needs. Enjoy the empowering sensation of strength and stability that these poses offer as you continue on your chair yoga journey.

3.4 Enhancing Balance and Coordination with Chair Yoga Flows

Chair yoga flows are sequences of gentle movements that help improve balance, coordination, and stability while seated or using a chair for support. These flows integrate breath, movement, and mindfulness to promote greater body awareness and enhance overall well-being. Incorporate these chair yoga flows into your practice to cultivate balance and coordination:

1. Seated Mountain Flow

- Sit tall on your chair with your feet flat on the floor and your hands resting on your thighs.
- Inhale as you reach your arms overhead, stretching upwards towards the sky.
- Exhale as you lower your arms back down to your sides, palms facing down.
- Repeat this flowing movement, synchronizing your breath with your movements.
- Focus on grounding down through your sit bones while reaching up through the crown of your head, finding a sense of stability and upliftment with each breath.

2. Seated Sun Salutation Flow

- Sit towards the front edge of your chair with your feet hip-width apart and your hands resting on your thighs.
- Inhale as you reach your arms overhead, lifting your chest and lengthening your spine.

- Exhale as you hinge forward at your hips and fold your torso over your thighs, reaching your hands towards your feet or the floor.

- Inhale as you lengthen your spine and lift your torso halfway up, coming into a flat back position.

- Exhale as you fold forward again, releasing any tension in your neck and shoulders.

- Inhale as you slowly roll back up to an upright position, stacking your vertebrae one by one.

- Repeat this flowing sequence, linking your breath with your movements, and maintaining a steady rhythm throughout.

3. Seated Warrior Flow

- Sit tall on your chair with your feet flat on the floor and your hands resting on your thighs.

- Inhale as you lift your arms overhead, reaching towards the sky.

- Exhale as you bring your right hand down to the side of your chair and lean to the right, stretching your left side body.

- Inhale as you return to center and reach your arms overhead again.

- Exhale as you bring your left hand down to the side of your chair and lean to the left, stretching your right side body.

- Continue flowing back and forth between these two movements, moving with your breath and maintaining a sense of balance and stability throughout.

4. Seated Tree Flow

- Sit tall on your chair with your feet flat on the floor and your hands resting on your thighs.

- Inhale as you lift your right foot off the floor and place the sole of your foot on the inside of your left thigh or calf, avoiding the knee.

- Exhale as you bring your hands together at your heart center in a prayer position.

- Inhale as you reach your arms overhead, growing tall like a tree.

- Exhale as you lower your arms back down to your sides and release your right foot back to the floor.

- Repeat this flow on the other side, lifting your left foot and placing it on the inside of your right thigh or calf.

- Continue flowing between these two sides, finding balance and stability in each variation of the pose.

5. Seated Balance Flow

- Sit tall on your chair with your feet flat on the floor and your hands resting on your thighs.

- Inhale as you lift your right foot off the floor and extend it forward, keeping your knee slightly bent.

- Exhale as you extend your right arm forward, reaching towards your toes.

"Zen Seats: Chair Yoga Mastery for Vibrant Seniors"

- Inhale as you return your right foot and arm back to the starting position.
- Repeat this flow on the other side, lifting your left foot and extending your left arm forward.
- Continue flowing between these two sides, focusing on maintaining a steady breath and finding stability in each balance variation.

6. Seated Twist Flow

- Sit tall on your chair with your feet flat on the floor and your hands resting on your thighs.
- Inhale as you lengthen your spine and lift your arms overhead.
- Exhale as you twist your torso to the right, bringing your left hand to the outside of your right thigh and your right hand to the back of your chair.
- Inhale as you lengthen your spine and lift your chest.
- Exhale as you deepen the twist, gazing over your right shoulder.
- Inhale as you return to center and reach your arms overhead again.
- Exhale as you twist to the left, repeating the sequence on the other side.
- Continue flowing between these two sides, moving with your breath and maintaining a sense of stability and ease in each twist.

7. Seated Warrior III Flow

- Sit tall on your chair with your feet flat on the floor and your hands resting on your thighs.
- Inhale as you lift your right leg off the floor and extend it straight back behind you, keeping your toes pointed and your hips square.
- Exhale as you hinge forward at your hips, lowering your torso towards your thighs and reaching your arms forward.
- Inhale as you lengthen your spine and lift your chest, finding a sense of balance and stability in the pose.
- Exhale as you return to the starting position, releasing your right foot back to the floor.
- Repeat this flow on the other side, lifting your left leg and extending it straight back behind you.
- Continue flowing between these two sides, moving with your breath and finding strength and stability in each variation of the pose.

Incorporate these chair yoga flows into your practice to enhance balance, coordination, and stability while seated or using a chair for support. Focus on moving mindfully, linking your breath with your movements, and maintaining a sense of ease and presence throughout. Enjoy the empowering sensation of balance and coordination that these flows offer as you continue on your chair yoga journey.

CHAPTER FOUR

4.1 Relaxation and Stress Relief Techniques

In today's fast-paced world, relaxation and stress relief techniques are essential for maintaining physical, mental, and emotional well-being. By incorporating a variety of relaxation techniques into your daily routine, you can effectively manage stress, promote relaxation, and cultivate a greater sense of inner peace and balance. Let's explore a comprehensive range of relaxation and stress relief techniques, leaving no stone unturned:

1. Deep Breathing Exercises:

- **Diaphragmatic Breathing:** Sit or lie down comfortably. Place one hand on your chest and the other on your abdomen. Inhale deeply through your nose, allowing your belly to rise as you fill your lungs with air. Exhale slowly through your mouth, feeling your belly fall. Repeat for several breaths, focusing on the rhythm of your breath and the sensation of expansion and release in your body.

- **4-7-8 Breathing:** Inhale deeply through your nose for a count of 4. Hold your breath for a count of 7. Exhale slowly through your mouth for a count of 8. Repeat this cycle for several rounds, allowing each exhalation to release tension and promote relaxation.

2. Progressive Muscle Relaxation (PMR):

- Start by sitting or lying down in a comfortable position.

"Zen Seats: Chair Yoga Mastery for Vibrant Seniors"

- Begin with your feet and work your way up through your body, systematically tensing and then releasing each muscle group. Hold the tension for a few seconds, then release and relax the muscles completely.
- Progressively move through your body, tensing and relaxing muscles in your legs, abdomen, chest, arms, shoulders, neck, and face.
- Pay attention to the sensations of relaxation as you release tension from each muscle group, allowing your body to sink deeper into a state of calm and ease.

3. Guided Imagery and Visualization:

- Close your eyes and imagine yourself in a peaceful, serene setting, such as a tranquil beach, a lush forest, or a cozy mountain cabin.
- Use all of your senses to create a vivid mental image of this relaxing environment. Notice the sights, sounds, smells, textures, and sensations around you.
- Allow yourself to fully immerse in the experience, letting go of any worries or concerns as you focus on the tranquility and beauty of your inner sanctuary.

4. Mindfulness Meditation:

- Find a quiet space where you can sit comfortably with your eyes closed.
- Bring your attention to your breath, noticing the sensation of each inhale and exhale.

- As thoughts, emotions, or sensations arise, simply observe them without judgment, allowing them to come and go like clouds passing through the sky.
- Continuously redirect your focus back to your breath whenever your mind begins to wander, cultivating a sense of presence and awareness in the present moment.

5. Yoga and Stretching:

- Practice gentle yoga poses or stretching exercises to release tension from your body and promote relaxation. Focus on slow, mindful movements that encourage deep breathing and connection with your body.
- Choose poses that target areas of tension or discomfort, such as forward folds, twists, hip openers, and gentle backbends.
- Pay attention to the sensations in your body as you move through each pose, honoring your limits and allowing yourself to find ease and comfort in each posture.

6. Massage and Self-Care:

- Treat yourself to a soothing massage or self-massage using gentle techniques such as kneading, stroking, and compression.
- Focus on areas of tension, such as your neck, shoulders, back, and feet, using your hands, fingers, or massage tools to release tight muscles and promote relaxation.

"Zen Seats: Chair Yoga Mastery for Vibrant Seniors"

- Incorporate other self-care practices into your routine, such as taking a warm bath, practicing aromatherapy with essential oils, or indulging in a calming cup of herbal tea.

7. Nature and Outdoor Activities:

- Spend time in nature to recharge and rejuvenate your spirit. Take a leisurely walk in the park, hike along a scenic trail, or simply sit and enjoy the beauty of the natural world.

- Engage in outdoor activities that bring you joy and relaxation, such as gardening, birdwatching, or picnicking in a peaceful setting.

- Connect with the sights, sounds, and sensations of the outdoors, allowing yourself to feel grounded and connected to the earth.

8. Creative Expression and Hobbies:

- Engage in creative activities that bring you joy and fulfillment, such as painting, drawing, writing, or crafting.

- Allow yourself to express your thoughts, feelings, and emotions through creative outlets, tapping into your inner creativity and imagination.

- Lose yourself in the process of creation, focusing on the present moment and allowing yourself to experience a sense of flow and relaxation.

9. Laughter and Humor:

- Surround yourself with people who bring joy and laughter into your life. Share lighthearted moments and humorous anecdotes with friends and loved ones.

- Watch a funny movie, read a humorous book, or listen to a comedy podcast to lift your spirits and lighten your mood.

- Allow yourself to laugh freely and fully, embracing the therapeutic power of laughter to reduce stress and promote relaxation.

10. Gratitude and Positive Affirmations:

- Cultivate an attitude of gratitude by reflecting on the things you're thankful for in your life. Take a few moments each day to acknowledge and appreciate the blessings, big and small, that surround you.

- Practice positive affirmations to reinforce feelings of self-worth, resilience, and optimism. Repeat affirmations such as "I am calm and centered," "I am worthy of love and happiness," or "I am capable of handling whatever comes my way."

- Focus on cultivating a mindset of abundance and positivity, allowing yourself to shift away from worry and fear towards gratitude and empowerment.

11. Social Connection and Support:

- Seek out social connection and support from friends, family, or support groups. Share your thoughts, feelings, and experiences with others who understand and empathize with you.

- Schedule regular social activities or outings that bring you joy and fulfillment, whether it's a coffee date with a friend, a game night with family, or a group fitness class.

- Lean on your support network during times of stress or difficulty, allowing yourself to receive comfort, encouragement, and assistance from those who care about you.

12. Mindful Movement and Exercise:

- Engage in mindful movement practices such as tai chi, qigong, or walking meditation to promote relaxation, focus, and presence.

- Incorporate regular exercise into your routine to reduce stress, boost mood, and improve overall well-being. Choose activities that you enjoy and that nourish your body and spirit.

- Pay attention to the sensations in your body as you move, honoring your body's needs and limitations while fostering a sense of connection and vitality.

13. Music and Sound Therapy:

- Listen to soothing music or nature sounds to create a calming atmosphere and promote relaxation. Experiment with different genres, artists, and playlists to find what resonates with you.

- Practice sound therapy techniques such as chanting, singing bowls, or guided audio meditations to quiet the mind, reduce stress, and promote inner peace.

- Allow yourself to immerse in the healing vibrations of sound, tuning into the rhythm and melody as you let go of tension and stress.

"Zen Seats: Chair Yoga Mastery for Vibrant Seniors"

14. Mindful Eating and Nutrition:

- Practice mindful eating by paying attention to the sensory experience of eating, including the taste, texture, aroma, and appearance of your food.

- Choose nourishing, whole foods that support your health and well-being, focusing on a balanced diet rich in fruits, vegetables, whole grains, lean proteins, and healthy fats.

- Avoid emotional eating or using food as a coping mechanism for stress. Instead, cultivate a healthy relationship with food by honoring your body's hunger and fullness cues and making conscious choices that support your overall health.

15. Sleep Hygiene and Relaxation Rituals:

- Prioritize quality sleep by establishing a consistent sleep schedule and creating a relaxing bedtime routine.

- Create a sleep-friendly environment by minimizing distractions, reducing noise and light, and ensuring your sleep space is comfortable and conducive to rest.

- Practice relaxation rituals before bed, such as gentle yoga stretches, deep breathing exercises, or reading a calming book, to signal to your body that it's time to unwind and prepare for sleep.

16. Professional Support and Therapy:

- Seek professional support from a therapist, counselor, or mental health professional if you're struggling to manage stress or cope with challenging emotions.

- Explore various therapeutic modalities and approaches, such as cognitive-behavioral therapy (CBT), mindfulness-based stress reduction (MBSR), or somatic experiencing, to find what resonates with you.

- Don't hesitate to reach out for help if you're experiencing significant distress or difficulty managing stress on your own. Remember that you're not alone, and support is available to help you navigate life's challenges.

Conclusion:

Incorporating a diverse range of relaxation and stress relief techniques into your daily life empowers you to effectively manage stress, promote relaxation, and enhance your overall well-being. Experiment with different techniques and practices to find what works best for you, and prioritize self-care as an essential part of your routine. By leaving no stone unturned and exploring a holistic approach to relaxation and stress relief, you can cultivate greater resilience, balance, and vitality in your life.

4.2 Guided Relaxation and Visualization Practices

Guided relaxation and visualization practices offer powerful tools for promoting relaxation, reducing stress, and enhancing overall well-being. By engaging your imagination and focusing your attention on calming imagery and sensations, you can create a profound sense of relaxation and inner peace. Let's explore a variety of guided relaxation and visualization practices, leaving no stone unturned:

1. Progressive Muscle Relaxation (PMR) Script:

- Begin by finding a comfortable position, either sitting or lying down, and take a few deep breaths to center yourself.

- Start by bringing your awareness to your feet. Take a deep breath in as you tense the muscles in your feet, and then exhale as you release the tension. Feel the sensation of relaxation spreading through your feet and into the rest of your body.

- Continue this process, gradually working your way up through your body, tensing and then releasing each muscle group, including your calves, thighs, abdomen, chest, arms, shoulders, neck, and face.

- As you release tension from each muscle group, imagine a wave of relaxation washing over you, melting away any stress or tension you may be holding onto.

- Take your time with each muscle group, allowing yourself to fully relax and let go with each exhale.

- Once you've completed the progressive muscle relaxation sequence, take a few moments to enjoy the deep sense of relaxation and peace that you've created.

2. Guided Imagery for Stress Relief:

- Close your eyes and take a few deep breaths to relax your body and quiet your mind.
- Imagine yourself in a peaceful and serene place, such as a beautiful beach, a tranquil forest, or a cozy mountain cabin.
- Use all of your senses to create a vivid mental image of this relaxing environment. Notice the sights, sounds, smells, textures, and sensations around you.
- Allow yourself to fully immerse in the experience, letting go of any worries or concerns as you bask in the tranquility and beauty of your inner sanctuary.
- Take a few moments to enjoy the peace and serenity of this imaginary place, allowing yourself to feel refreshed and rejuvenated.

3. Visualization for Confidence and Empowerment:

- Close your eyes and take a few deep breaths to center yourself.
- Imagine yourself stepping into a room filled with light and energy. This room represents your inner strength, confidence, and power.
- Visualize yourself standing tall and strong, radiating confidence and self-assurance. Feel the energy and

power coursing through your body, filling you with a sense of empowerment.

- Take a moment to connect with this feeling of confidence and strength, allowing it to flow through you and uplift you in every way.

- Carry this sense of empowerment with you throughout your day, knowing that you have the inner strength and resilience to overcome any challenges that come your way.

4. Guided Relaxation for Sleep:

- Find a comfortable position in bed and take a few deep breaths to relax your body and mind.

- Close your eyes and imagine yourself in a peaceful and cozy bedroom, surrounded by soft blankets and pillows.

- Visualize a warm and comforting light surrounding you, enveloping you in a sense of safety and security.

- As you breathe deeply, imagine each inhale bringing relaxation and calmness into your body, and each exhale releasing any tension or stress.

- Allow yourself to sink deeper into a state of relaxation with each breath, feeling yourself becoming more and more drowsy and ready for sleep.

- Continue to focus on your breath and the soothing imagery until you drift off into a peaceful and restful sleep.

5. Guided Meditation for Inner Peace:

- Find a comfortable seated position and close your eyes.
- Take a few deep breaths to center yourself and relax your body and mind.
- Imagine a ball of warm, golden light glowing at the center of your chest. This light represents your inner peace and serenity.
- With each inhale, imagine this light expanding and filling your entire body, bathing every cell in its warm and comforting glow.
- With each exhale, feel any tension or stress melting away, leaving you feeling calm, centered, and at peace.
- Allow yourself to bask in this feeling of inner peace for as long as you like, knowing that you can return to this state of calm and tranquility whenever you need it.

Conclusion:

Guided relaxation and visualization practices offer powerful techniques for promoting relaxation, reducing stress, and cultivating a greater sense of well-being. By engaging your imagination and focusing your attention on calming imagery and sensations, you can create a profound sense of relaxation and inner peace. Experiment with different guided scripts and practices to find what resonates with you, and incorporate these techniques into your daily routine to support your mental, emotional, and physical health. With practice and patience, you can harness the transformative power of guided relaxation and visualization to create a life filled with peace, balance, and joy.

4.3 Breathing Exercises for Calmness and Clarity

Breathing exercises are potent tools for achieving a state of calmness and clarity in the midst of life's challenges. By harnessing the power of your breath, you can regulate your nervous system, reduce stress, and cultivate mental clarity. Let's explore a comprehensive range of breathing exercises, ensuring no stone is left unturned in your pursuit of inner peace and clarity:

1. Diaphragmatic Breathing (Belly Breathing):

- Find a comfortable seated position or lie down on your back with your knees bent and your feet flat on the floor.

- Place one hand on your chest and the other on your abdomen.

- Inhale deeply through your nose, allowing your belly to rise as you fill your lungs with air. Feel your abdomen expand outward, pushing against your hand.

- Exhale slowly through your mouth, allowing your belly to fall as you release the air from your lungs. Feel your abdomen contract inward.

- Continue this deep belly breathing for several minutes, focusing on the sensation of your breath filling and emptying your lungs. Notice how each breath brings a sense of calmness and clarity to your mind.

2. Box Breathing (Square Breathing):

- Sit comfortably in a quiet space and close your eyes.
- Inhale deeply through your nose for a count of four, filling your lungs with air and expanding your belly.
- Hold your breath for a count of four, maintaining a sense of stillness and presence.
- Exhale slowly through your mouth for a count of four, emptying your lungs completely and allowing your belly to deflate.
- Hold your breath again for a count of four before beginning the next inhalation.
- Repeat this box breathing pattern for several rounds, allowing each breath to anchor you in the present moment and bring clarity to your mind.

3. Alternate Nostril Breathing (Nadi Shodhana):

- Sit comfortably with your spine tall and your shoulders relaxed.
- Place your left hand on your left knee with your palm facing upward.
- Bring your right hand to your face and use your thumb to close your right nostril.
- Inhale deeply through your left nostril, filling your lungs with air.

- Close your left nostril with your ring finger and release your thumb from your right nostril.
- Exhale slowly through your right nostril, emptying your lungs completely.
- Inhale deeply through your right nostril.
- Close your right nostril with your thumb and release your ring finger from your left nostril.
- Exhale slowly through your left nostril.
- Continue this alternate nostril breathing pattern for several rounds, focusing on the smooth and steady flow of your breath and the sense of balance and clarity it brings to your mind.

4. 4-7-8 Breathing (Relaxing Breath):

- Sit comfortably or lie down in a quiet space.
- Place the tip of your tongue against the roof of your mouth behind your front teeth.
- Inhale quietly through your nose for a count of four, allowing your belly to expand with each breath.
- Hold your breath for a count of seven.
- Exhale forcefully through your mouth for a count of eight, making a whooshing sound as you release the air from your lungs.
- Repeat this 4-7-8 breathing pattern for several rounds, allowing each exhalation to release tension and promote relaxation in your body and mind.

5. Lion's Breath (Simhasana Pranayama):

- Kneel on the floor with your knees hip-width apart and your buttocks resting on your heels.
- Place your hands on your thighs with your fingers spread wide.
- Inhale deeply through your nose, filling your lungs with air.
- Exhale forcefully through your mouth, sticking out your tongue and roaring like a lion. Feel the breath leaving your body with power and intensity.
- Repeat this lion's breath for several rounds, allowing each exhalation to release pent-up energy and tension from your body and mind.

6. Humming Bee Breath (Bhramari Pranayama):

- Sit comfortably with your spine tall and your shoulders relaxed.
- Close your eyes and take a few deep breaths to center yourself.
- Place your index fingers on the cartilage between your cheeks and ears, lightly pressing down to close off your ears.
- Inhale deeply through your nose.
- Exhale slowly and deeply, making a low-pitched humming sound like that of a bee. Feel the vibration of the sound reverberating throughout your head and body.

- Continue this humming bee breath for several rounds, allowing each exhalation to calm your nervous system and bring clarity to your mind.

7. Sama Vritti (Equal Breathing):

- Sit comfortably with your spine tall and your shoulders relaxed.
- Inhale slowly and deeply through your nose for a count of four.
- Exhale slowly and completely through your nose for a count of four.
- Continue this equal breathing pattern for several rounds, maintaining a smooth and steady rhythm with each inhalation and exhalation.
- As you breathe, imagine your mind becoming calmer and clearer with each breath, free from distractions and worries.

Conclusion:

Breathing exercises offer a myriad of benefits for promoting calmness and clarity in your mind and body. By incorporating these techniques into your daily routine, you can regulate your nervous system, reduce stress, and cultivate a greater sense of mental clarity and focus. Experiment with different breathing exercises to find what works best for you, and make them a regular part of your self-care toolkit. With practice and consistency, you can harness the transformative power of your breath to achieve a state of calmness and clarity in any situation life throws your way.

4.4 Using Props and Modifications for Comfort and Support

In the practice of yoga, props and modifications play a crucial role in ensuring comfort, safety, and accessibility for practitioners of all levels and abilities. By incorporating props such as blocks, straps, blankets, bolsters, and chairs, individuals can adapt poses to suit their unique needs, limitations, and body types. Let's explore how props and modifications can be utilized effectively to enhance comfort and provide support in yoga practice, leaving no stone unturned in our exploration:

1. Blocks:

- **Purpose:** Blocks are versatile props used to modify poses by providing support, stability, and extension. They can be used to bring the floor closer to the practitioner, reduce strain, and assist in maintaining proper alignment.

- **Examples of Use:**
    - Placing blocks under the hands in standing forward bends to bring the floor closer and maintain a straight spine.
    - Using blocks under the hips in seated poses to elevate the pelvis and ease discomfort.
    - Supporting the head in supported fish pose by placing a block under the upper back and head.

2. Straps:

- **Purpose:** Straps are excellent tools for increasing flexibility, extending reach, and enhancing alignment in yoga poses. They can be used to bridge the gap between the hands and feet, allowing practitioners to access deeper stretches safely and effectively.

- **Examples of Use:**

    - Using a strap to extend the arms in seated forward bends or seated twists, providing leverage and support for deeper stretches.

    - Wrapping a strap around the feet in seated forward folds to maintain alignment and prevent rounding of the spine.

    - Holding onto a strap in standing poses such as dancer's pose or half moon pose to assist in balance and stability.

3. Blankets:

- **Purpose:** Blankets offer padding, cushioning, and warmth, making them valuable props for enhancing comfort and relaxation in yoga practice. They can be used to support the body in reclined poses, provide extra padding under sensitive joints, and create a cozy environment for meditation and relaxation.

- **Examples of Use:**

    - Folding blankets to create support under the knees or hips in reclined poses such as supported bridge pose or legs up the wall pose.

"Zen Seats: Chair Yoga Mastery for Vibrant Seniors"

- Rolling blankets to place under the spine in restorative poses such as supported fish pose or supported supine twist.
- Using blankets as props for seated meditation or pranayama practices to provide warmth and comfort.

4. Bolsters:

- **Purpose:** Bolsters are large, firm cushions designed to provide support and relaxation in restorative yoga poses. They offer gentle elevation and padding, allowing practitioners to fully relax into poses without strain or discomfort.

- **Examples of Use:**
    - Placing a bolster under the knees in savasana (corpse pose) to release tension in the lower back and legs.
    - Using a bolster to support the spine in reclining bound angle pose, allowing the chest to open and the shoulders to relax.
    - Resting the forehead on a bolster in child's pose to promote relaxation and surrender.

5. Chairs:

- **Purpose:** Chairs are valuable props for individuals with limited mobility, balance issues, or injuries, providing stability, support, and accessibility in yoga practice. They can be used to modify standing, seated, and reclined poses, making yoga accessible to a wide range of practitioners.

- **Examples of Use:**
    - Using a chair for support in standing poses such as mountain pose or warrior poses to maintain balance and stability.
    - Sitting on a chair for seated poses such as seated forward bends or twists to reduce strain on the lower back and hips.
    - Using a chair as a prop for restorative poses such as supported shoulder stand or legs up the wall pose to provide support and relaxation.

6. Modifications for Special Populations:
- **Purpose:** Modifications are essential for accommodating special populations such as seniors, pregnant individuals, or individuals with physical limitations or injuries. By adapting poses and sequences to suit the needs of these populations, yoga can be made safe, accessible, and beneficial for all.
- **Examples of Use:**
    - Offering seated variations of standing poses for seniors or individuals with limited mobility, focusing on gentle movement and breath awareness.
    - Providing prenatal modifications for pregnant individuals, including props such as bolsters, blankets, and chairs to support the body and accommodate the growing belly.

- Offering modifications for individuals with injuries or physical limitations, such as using props to reduce strain and support proper alignment in poses.

Conclusion:

Props and modifications are indispensable tools for enhancing comfort, safety, and accessibility in yoga practice. By utilizing props such as blocks, straps, blankets, bolsters, and chairs, practitioners can adapt poses to suit their unique needs, limitations, and body types. Modifications are essential for accommodating special populations and ensuring that yoga is inclusive and beneficial for all individuals. By embracing props and modifications, yoga practitioners can cultivate a practice that is supportive, nourishing, and transformative, leaving no stone unturned in their journey towards health, well-being, and self-discovery.

CHAPTER FIVE

5.1 CHAIR YOGA FOR EVERYDAY LIFE

Chair yoga offers a gentle and accessible approach to yoga practice that can be integrated seamlessly into everyday life. Whether you're at home, at work, or traveling, chair yoga provides an opportunity to cultivate mindfulness, relieve tension, and promote overall well-being without the need for a yoga mat or specialized equipment. Let's explore how chair yoga can enhance your everyday life, covering its benefits, techniques, and practical applications:

Benefits of Chair Yoga:

1. **Accessibility:** Chair yoga is accessible to individuals of all ages, fitness levels, and physical abilities. It can be adapted to suit individual needs and limitations, making it ideal for seniors, those with mobility issues, or individuals recovering from injuries.

2. **Convenience:** Chair yoga can be practiced anywhere, anytime, using a sturdy chair as the primary prop. Whether you're at home, at the office, or traveling, you can easily incorporate chair yoga into your daily routine without the need for a large practice space or specialized equipment.

3. **Stress Reduction:** Chair yoga offers gentle movements, breath awareness, and relaxation techniques that help reduce stress and promote relaxation. By incorporating mindfulness practices into your day, you can better manage stress, improve mood, and enhance overall well-being.

"Zen Seats: Chair Yoga Mastery for Vibrant Seniors"

4. **Improved Flexibility and Mobility:** Chair yoga includes a variety of gentle stretches and movements that help improve flexibility, mobility, and range of motion. Regular practice can alleviate stiffness, reduce joint pain, and increase overall comfort and ease of movement.

5. **Posture Support:** Many chair yoga poses focus on alignment, core stability, and postural awareness, helping to improve posture and alleviate common issues such as back pain, neck tension, and shoulder tightness.

6. **Mind-Body Connection:** Chair yoga encourages a deepening of the mind-body connection through conscious movement, breath work, and relaxation techniques. By tuning into your body's sensations and focusing your attention inward, you can cultivate greater awareness, presence, and self-awareness.

Techniques for Chair Yoga Practice:

1. **Seated Breathing Exercises:** Begin your chair yoga practice with simple breathing exercises to center your mind and body. Practice deep belly breathing, equal breathing, or guided breath awareness to promote relaxation and focus.

2. **Gentle Stretches and Movements:** Incorporate gentle stretches and movements to release tension, improve flexibility, and promote circulation. Focus on areas of the body that feel tight or tense, such as the neck, shoulders, spine, hips, and legs.

3. **Chair Yoga Poses:** Explore a variety of seated and standing yoga poses that can be adapted to the chair.

"Zen Seats: Chair Yoga Mastery for Vibrant Seniors"

Include poses such as seated forward fold, seated twist, seated cat-cow stretch, chair mountain pose, chair warrior pose, and chair pigeon pose.

4. **Mindfulness Meditation:** Integrate mindfulness meditation practices into your chair yoga routine to cultivate presence, awareness, and inner peace. Practice seated meditation, guided visualization, or body scan meditation to quiet the mind and reduce stress.

5. **Relaxation Techniques:** Conclude your chair yoga practice with relaxation techniques to promote deep relaxation and rejuvenation. Practice progressive muscle relaxation, guided relaxation, or yoga nidra to release tension and restore balance.

Practical Applications in Everyday Life:

1. **At Home:** Practice chair yoga at home as part of your morning routine, during breaks throughout the day, or as a wind-down activity in the evening. Use a comfortable chair in a quiet space where you can focus and relax.

2. **At Work:** Incorporate chair yoga into your workday to relieve stress, improve focus, and boost productivity. Take short breaks to practice seated stretches, breathing exercises, or mindfulness meditation at your desk or in a quiet corner of the office.

3. **While Traveling:** Use chair yoga as a convenient way to stay grounded and centered while traveling. Practice seated stretches, breathing techniques, and mindfulness exercises during long flights, layovers,

or road trips to reduce stiffness and promote relaxation.

4. **For Seniors:** Chair yoga is particularly beneficial for seniors as it provides a safe and accessible way to stay active, mobile, and healthy. Seniors can practice chair yoga in community centers, retirement homes, or in the comfort of their own homes with the support of a qualified instructor or video guidance.

5. **For Rehabilitation:** Chair yoga can be used as part of a rehabilitation program for individuals recovering from injuries, surgeries, or chronic health conditions. It offers gentle movement, pain relief, and emotional support during the healing process, helping individuals regain strength, flexibility, and confidence.

Conclusion:

Chair yoga offers a multitude of benefits for enhancing everyday life, from stress reduction and improved flexibility to enhanced mindfulness and well-being. By incorporating chair yoga into your daily routine, you can experience greater comfort, relaxation, and vitality in mind, body, and spirit. Whether you're at home, at work, or on the go, chair yoga provides a convenient and accessible way to nurture your physical, mental, and emotional health, leaving you feeling grounded, centered, and rejuvenated in every aspect of your life.

5.2 Integrating Chair Yoga into Daily Routines: A Comprehensive Guide

Chair yoga offers a convenient and accessible way to incorporate the benefits of yoga into your daily routine, regardless of your schedule, space constraints, or physical limitations. By integrating chair yoga into your daily activities, you can enhance flexibility, reduce stress, and promote overall well-being without the need for a yoga mat or specialized equipment. Let's explore how you can seamlessly weave chair yoga into your daily routines, covering morning, daytime, and evening practices:

Morning Routine:

1. **Wake-Up Stretch:** Start your day with a gentle wake-up stretch routine using your chair. Sit comfortably and stretch your arms overhead, lengthening through your spine and reaching towards the ceiling. Hold for a few breaths, then release and repeat several times.

2. **Seated Sun Salutations:** Practice a modified version of sun salutations while seated in your chair. Inhale as you reach your arms up, exhale as you fold forward, and inhale to lift halfway. Continue flowing through the sequence, linking your breath with movement to wake up your body and mind.

3. **Mindful Breathing:** Take a few moments to practice mindful breathing before starting your day. Sit comfortably in your chair, close your eyes, and focus on your breath. Inhale deeply through your nose, exhale fully through your mouth, and repeat for several breaths to center yourself and cultivate presence.

"Zen Seats: Chair Yoga Mastery for Vibrant Seniors"

Daytime Routine:

1. **Desk Yoga Breaks:** Incorporate short chair yoga breaks throughout your workday to relieve tension and boost energy. Practice seated stretches, shoulder rolls, neck rotations, and wrist exercises at your desk to release stiffness and improve circulation.

2. **Chair Yoga at Lunchtime:** Use your lunch break as an opportunity to practice chair yoga for relaxation and rejuvenation. Find a quiet space away from your desk, sit comfortably in your chair, and practice gentle stretches, breathing exercises, or mindfulness meditation to refresh your body and mind.

3. **Stress Reduction Techniques:** Whenever you feel stressed or overwhelmed during the day, take a moment to practice stress reduction techniques with your chair yoga practice. Close your eyes, take a few deep breaths, and engage in calming poses or relaxation exercises to promote relaxation and clarity.

Evening Routine:

1. **Evening Wind-Down:** Wind down at the end of the day with a soothing chair yoga practice to relax your body and prepare for sleep. Practice gentle stretches, restorative poses, and relaxation techniques to release tension and calm your nervous system before bedtime.

2. **Bedtime Yoga Ritual:** Create a bedtime yoga ritual using your chair as a support prop. Sit in your chair and practice slow, mindful movements, such as gentle twists, side stretches, and forward bends, to

ease tension and promote relaxation. End your practice with a few minutes of deep breathing and meditation to quiet your mind and prepare for sleep.

3. **Mindful Reflection:** Before going to bed, take a few moments to reflect on your day with mindfulness. Sit quietly in your chair, close your eyes, and review the events of the day with compassion and acceptance. Practice gratitude for the positive moments and let go of any worries or concerns as you prepare for restful sleep.

Additional Tips:

1. **Set Reminders:** Use alarms, calendar notifications, or mindfulness apps to remind yourself to integrate chair yoga into your daily routines. Set aside dedicated time for practice and prioritize your well-being throughout the day.

2. **Be Flexible:** Be flexible and adaptable with your chair yoga practice, especially on busy days or during hectic periods. Even a few minutes of mindful breathing or gentle stretching can make a significant difference in how you feel.

3. **Listen to Your Body:** Listen to your body's cues and adjust your chair yoga practice accordingly. If you experience discomfort or pain during a pose, modify or skip it altogether. Honor your body's needs and practice self-care with kindness and compassion.

4. **Experiment and Explore:** Experiment with different chair yoga poses, sequences, and techniques to find what works best for you. Explore

guided videos, books, or online resources for inspiration and guidance in your practice.

Conclusion:

Integrating chair yoga into your daily routines offers a practical and sustainable way to prioritize your physical, mental, and emotional well-being. By incorporating mindful movement, breath awareness, and relaxation techniques into your morning, daytime, and evening activities, you can cultivate a sense of balance, ease, and vitality in every aspect of your life. Whether you're at home, at work, or on the go, chair yoga provides a valuable opportunity to nurture yourself and enhance your overall quality of life.

5.3 Integrating Chair Yoga into Daily Routines: A Comprehensive Guide

Chair yoga offers a convenient and accessible way to incorporate the benefits of yoga into your daily routine, regardless of your schedule, space constraints, or physical limitations. By integrating chair yoga into your daily activities, you can enhance flexibility, reduce stress, and promote overall well-being without the need for a yoga mat or specialized equipment. Let's explore how you can seamlessly weave chair yoga into your daily routines, covering morning, daytime, and evening practices:

Morning Routine:

1. **Wake-Up Stretch:** Start your day with a gentle wake-up stretch routine using your chair. Sit comfortably and stretch your arms overhead, lengthening through your spine and reaching towards

"Zen Seats: Chair Yoga Mastery for Vibrant Seniors"

the ceiling. Hold for a few breaths, then release and repeat several times.

2. **Seated Sun Salutations:** Practice a modified version of sun salutations while seated in your chair. Inhale as you reach your arms up, exhale as you fold forward, and inhale to lift halfway. Continue flowing through the sequence, linking your breath with movement to wake up your body and mind.

3. **Mindful Breathing:** Take a few moments to practice mindful breathing before starting your day. Sit comfortably in your chair, close your eyes, and focus on your breath. Inhale deeply through your nose, exhale fully through your mouth, and repeat for several breaths to center yourself and cultivate presence.

Daytime Routine:

1. **Desk Yoga Breaks:** Incorporate short chair yoga breaks throughout your workday to relieve tension and boost energy. Practice seated stretches, shoulder rolls, neck rotations, and wrist exercises at your desk to release stiffness and improve circulation.

2. **Chair Yoga at Lunchtime:** Use your lunch break as an opportunity to practice chair yoga for relaxation and rejuvenation. Find a quiet space away from your desk, sit comfortably in your chair, and practice gentle stretches, breathing exercises, or mindfulness meditation to refresh your body and mind.

3. **Stress Reduction Techniques:** Whenever you feel stressed or overwhelmed during the day, take a moment to practice stress reduction techniques with

your chair yoga practice. Close your eyes, take a few deep breaths, and engage in calming poses or relaxation exercises to promote relaxation and clarity.

Evening Routine:

1. **Evening Wind-Down:** Wind down at the end of the day with a soothing chair yoga practice to relax your body and prepare for sleep. Practice gentle stretches, restorative poses, and relaxation techniques to release tension and calm your nervous system before bedtime.

2. **Bedtime Yoga Ritual:** Create a bedtime yoga ritual using your chair as a support prop. Sit in your chair and practice slow, mindful movements, such as gentle twists, side stretches, and forward bends, to ease tension and promote relaxation. End your practice with a few minutes of deep breathing and meditation to quiet your mind and prepare for sleep.

3. **Mindful Reflection:** Before going to bed, take a few moments to reflect on your day with mindfulness. Sit quietly in your chair, close your eyes, and review the events of the day with compassion and acceptance. Practice gratitude for the positive moments and let go of any worries or concerns as you prepare for restful sleep.

Additional Tips:

1. **Set Reminders:** Use alarms, calendar notifications, or mindfulness apps to remind yourself to integrate chair yoga into your daily routines. Set aside

dedicated time for practice and prioritize your well-being throughout the day.

2. **Be Flexible:** Be flexible and adaptable with your chair yoga practice, especially on busy days or during hectic periods. Even a few minutes of mindful breathing or gentle stretching can make a significant difference in how you feel.

3. **Listen to Your Body:** Listen to your body's cues and adjust your chair yoga practice accordingly. If you experience discomfort or pain during a pose, modify or skip it altogether. Honor your body's needs and practice self-care with kindness and compassion.

4. **Experiment and Explore:** Experiment with different chair yoga poses, sequences, and techniques to find what works best for you. Explore guided videos, books, or online resources for inspiration and guidance in your practice.

Conclusion:

Integrating chair yoga into your daily routines offers a practical and sustainable way to prioritize your physical, mental, and emotional well-being. By incorporating mindful movement, breath awareness, and relaxation techniques into your morning, daytime, and evening activities, you can cultivate a sense of balance, ease, and vitality in every aspect of your life. Whether you're at home, at work, or on the go, chair yoga provides a valuable opportunity to nurture yourself and enhance your overall quality of life.

5.4 Mindful Movement for Improved Focus and Energy

In today's fast-paced world, finding moments of focus and sustaining energy throughout the day can be challenging. Mindful movement offers a powerful solution, allowing you to cultivate presence, enhance concentration, and boost vitality through intentional movement and breath awareness. Let's delve into the practice of mindful movement and explore how it can help you improve focus and energy levels:

Understanding Mindful Movement:

Mindful movement involves bringing conscious awareness to every aspect of movement, including posture, alignment, breath, and intention. It encourages a deepening of the mind-body connection, fostering greater awareness of physical sensations, thoughts, and emotions as you move through different activities. By practicing mindful movement, you can cultivate a sense of presence, reduce distractions, and enhance your ability to engage fully in the present moment.

Benefits of Mindful Movement for Improved Focus and Energy:

1. **Increased Concentration:** Mindful movement requires focused attention on the present moment, helping to sharpen your concentration and reduce mental chatter. By directing your awareness to the sensations of movement and breath, you can anchor your attention and stay centered amidst distractions.

2. **Enhanced Mind-Body Connection:** Mindful movement encourages a deeper connection between the mind and body, allowing you to move with

greater awareness and intention. By tuning into the physical sensations of movement, you can cultivate a sense of embodiment and presence, fostering a holistic sense of well-being.

3. **Stress Reduction:** Mindful movement promotes relaxation and stress reduction by activating the body's relaxation response and calming the nervous system. By moving mindfully and focusing on the breath, you can soothe the mind, release tension, and cultivate a sense of ease and calmness.

4. **Improved Energy Levels:** Engaging in mindful movement can boost energy levels by increasing circulation, oxygenating the body, and invigorating the mind. By moving with intention and awareness, you can stimulate the flow of vital energy throughout the body, leaving you feeling refreshed and revitalized.

5. **Enhanced Productivity:** Mindful movement can enhance productivity by improving mental clarity, creativity, and problem-solving abilities. By taking short movement breaks throughout the day, you can reset your focus, re-energize your body, and approach tasks with renewed vigor and clarity.

Practicing Mindful Movement:

1. **Body Scan Meditation:** Begin by bringing your attention to different parts of your body, starting from your toes and gradually moving up to your head. Notice any sensations, tension, or areas of discomfort, and breathe into those areas with gentle awareness. This practice helps to release tension, promote relaxation, and cultivate body awareness.

"Zen Seats: Chair Yoga Mastery for Vibrant Seniors"

2. **Mindful Walking:** Take a short walk outdoors or indoors while focusing your attention on the sensation of each step. Notice the contact of your feet with the ground, the rhythm of your breath, and the sights and sounds around you. Allow yourself to fully immerse in the experience of walking, letting go of distractions and cultivating presence.

3. **Yoga Flow:** Practice a series of yoga poses or movements with mindful awareness, paying attention to your breath, alignment, and sensations as you move through each posture. Flow seamlessly from one pose to the next, linking movement with breath to create a fluid and meditative practice.

4. **Tai Chi or Qigong:** Engage in gentle martial arts practices such as tai chi or qigong, which emphasize slow, deliberate movements coordinated with deep breathing and focused attention. These practices promote balance, flexibility, and inner calmness, fostering a sense of flow and harmony in movement.

5. **Desk Stretches:** Incorporate short movement breaks into your workday with simple stretches and movements at your desk. Focus on areas of tension such as the neck, shoulders, and hips, and perform gentle stretches to release tightness and improve circulation.

"Zen Seats: Chair Yoga Mastery for Vibrant Seniors"

Tips for Incorporating Mindful Movement into Your Routine:

1. **Set Intentions:** Start each mindful movement practice with a clear intention or goal in mind, whether it's to cultivate focus, release tension, or increase energy levels. Setting intentions helps to guide your practice and enhance its effectiveness.

2. **Practice Regularly:** Make mindful movement a regular part of your daily routine by scheduling time for practice each day. Whether it's a short session in the morning, a movement break during the day, or an evening practice to wind down, consistency is key to experiencing the benefits of mindful movement.

3. **Listen to Your Body:** Pay attention to your body's cues and limitations during mindful movement practice, and modify poses or movements as needed to suit your individual needs. Honor your body's wisdom and practice self-care with compassion and kindness.

4. **Stay Present:** Keep your attention anchored in the present moment during mindful movement practice by focusing on the sensations of movement and breath. Let go of distractions, worries, and judgments, and simply be with the experience as it unfolds.

5. **Express Gratitude:** Cultivate a sense of gratitude for your body and its ability to move, breathe, and experience the world around you. Approach mindful movement practice with an attitude of appreciation and curiosity, and embrace each moment as an opportunity for growth and exploration.

"Zen Seats: Chair Yoga Mastery for Vibrant Seniors"

Conclusion:

Mindful movement offers a powerful pathway to improved focus, energy, and well-being by cultivating presence, enhancing body awareness, and reducing stress. By incorporating mindful movement practices into your daily routine, you can tap into a profound sense of vitality, clarity, and aliveness, allowing you to engage fully in the present moment and live with greater intention and purpose. Whether you choose to practice yoga, tai chi, walking meditation, or simple desk stretches, the key is to approach movement with mindful awareness, bringing attention, intention, and presence to each moment.

CHAPTER SIX

6.1 CHAIR YOGA FOR SPECIFIC HEALTH CONCERNS

Chair yoga is a versatile and accessible practice that can be adapted to address a wide range of health concerns, including physical limitations, chronic conditions, and age-related issues. By incorporating gentle movements, breath awareness, and relaxation techniques, chair yoga offers a holistic approach to wellness that can complement traditional medical treatments and support overall health and well-being. Let's explore how chair yoga can be tailored to address specific health concerns:

1. Arthritis:

- Chair yoga offers gentle movements and stretches that can help alleviate stiffness, reduce pain, and improve joint mobility for individuals with arthritis.

- Focus on gentle range-of-motion exercises, such as wrist circles, ankle rolls, and shoulder rotations, to lubricate the joints and increase flexibility.

- Incorporate breath awareness and relaxation techniques to reduce stress and tension, which can exacerbate arthritis symptoms.

2. Osteoporosis:

- Chair yoga can help individuals with osteoporosis improve balance, coordination, and bone density while reducing the risk of fractures.

- Include weight-bearing exercises such as seated leg lifts, heel raises, and seated squats to strengthen bones and muscles.
- Emphasize gentle backbends and spinal twists to promote spinal health and maintain mobility in the spine.

3. Chronic Pain:

- Chair yoga provides a gentle and low-impact way to manage chronic pain conditions such as fibromyalgia, back pain, and neuropathy.
- Focus on gentle stretches and movements that target areas of tension and discomfort, such as the neck, shoulders, lower back, and hips.
- Incorporate relaxation techniques such as deep breathing, guided imagery, and progressive muscle relaxation to reduce pain perception and promote relaxation.

4. Stress and Anxiety:

- Chair yoga offers a calming and grounding practice that can help reduce stress and anxiety levels by activating the body's relaxation response.
- Include slow, mindful movements such as gentle stretches, flowing sequences, and breath awareness exercises to soothe the nervous system and promote relaxation.
- Integrate meditation and mindfulness practices into your chair yoga routine to cultivate present-moment awareness and reduce rumination and worry.

5. Cardiovascular Health:

- Chair yoga can be beneficial for individuals with cardiovascular issues by improving circulation, reducing blood pressure, and promoting heart health.

- Include gentle aerobic exercises such as seated marching, arm circles, and seated twists to increase heart rate and improve cardiovascular fitness.

- Incorporate relaxation techniques such as deep breathing and guided visualization to promote relaxation and reduce stress, which can benefit overall heart health.

6. Respiratory Conditions:

- Chair yoga can help individuals with respiratory conditions such as asthma, COPD, and bronchitis improve lung function, increase oxygenation, and reduce symptoms.

- Focus on deep breathing exercises such as diaphragmatic breathing, pursed lip breathing, and alternate nostril breathing to strengthen respiratory muscles and improve lung capacity.

- Incorporate gentle chest opening poses and seated backbends to promote expansion of the chest and improve breathing mechanics.

7. Diabetes:

- Chair yoga can be a beneficial addition to diabetes management by promoting blood sugar regulation, reducing stress levels, and improving circulation.

"Zen Seats: Chair Yoga Mastery for Vibrant Seniors"

- Include gentle aerobic exercises such as seated marching, leg lifts, and arm movements to promote circulation and increase insulin sensitivity.
- Integrate relaxation techniques such as deep breathing, progressive muscle relaxation, and guided imagery to reduce stress and promote overall well-being.

8. Age-Related Concerns:

- Chair yoga is well-suited for older adults as it provides support, stability, and accessibility while addressing age-related concerns such as balance issues, mobility limitations, and decreased flexibility.
- Focus on gentle movements and stretches that improve joint mobility, muscle strength, and flexibility while reducing the risk of falls and injuries.
- Incorporate relaxation techniques such as deep breathing, mindfulness meditation, and gentle movement sequences to promote relaxation, reduce stress, and support overall well-being.

Conclusion:

Chair yoga offers a gentle and accessible approach to addressing a wide range of health concerns, making it suitable for individuals of all ages and abilities. Whether you're managing chronic pain, seeking stress relief, or looking to improve cardiovascular health, chair yoga can be tailored to meet your specific needs and support your overall well-being. By incorporating gentle movements, breath awareness, and relaxation techniques into your daily routine, you can experience the transformative benefits of chair yoga and enhance your quality of life. It's important to consult with a healthcare professional before starting any new exercise program, especially if you have underlying health concerns or medical conditions.

6.2 Managing Arthritis and Joint Pain with Chair Yoga

Arthritis and joint pain can significantly impact mobility, comfort, and quality of life. Chair yoga offers a gentle and accessible way to manage arthritis symptoms, improve joint mobility, and reduce pain while promoting overall well-being. By incorporating gentle movements, breath awareness, and relaxation techniques, chair yoga can provide relief and support for individuals living with arthritis. Let's explore how chair yoga can be used to manage arthritis and joint pain effectively:

Understanding Arthritis:

Arthritis is a common condition characterized by inflammation and stiffness in the joints, which can result in pain, swelling, and limited mobility. There are several types of arthritis, including osteoarthritis, rheumatoid arthritis, and psoriatic arthritis, each with its own unique symptoms and challenges. While there is no cure for arthritis, managing symptoms and maintaining joint health through lifestyle modifications, including exercise, can help improve overall function and quality of life.

"Zen Seats: Chair Yoga Mastery for Vibrant Seniors"

Benefits of Chair Yoga for Arthritis:

1. **Gentle Movement:** Chair yoga offers gentle movements and stretches that can help improve joint mobility, reduce stiffness, and increase flexibility without putting undue stress on the joints.

2. **Strengthening Muscles:** Chair yoga poses can help strengthen the muscles surrounding the joints, providing support and stability and reducing the risk of injury.

3. **Pain Relief:** Chair yoga promotes relaxation and stress reduction, which can help alleviate pain and discomfort associated with arthritis.

4. **Improved Range of Motion:** Regular practice of chair yoga can help improve range of motion in the joints, allowing for better flexibility and ease of movement.

5. **Enhanced Mind-Body Connection:** Chair yoga encourages mindfulness and body awareness, allowing individuals to tune into their bodies and better manage arthritis symptoms.

Chair Yoga Poses for Arthritis:

1. **Seated Cat-Cow Stretch:** Sit comfortably in your chair with your feet flat on the floor. Inhale as you arch your back and lift your chest (cow pose), then exhale as you round your spine and tuck your chin to your chest (cat pose). Repeat several times, moving with your breath.

2. **Seated Twist:** Sit upright in your chair with your feet flat on the floor. Inhale to lengthen your spine, then

"Zen Seats: Chair Yoga Mastery for Vibrant Seniors"

exhale as you twist to the right, placing your left hand on the outside of your right knee and your right hand on the back of the chair. Hold for a few breaths, then repeat on the other side.

3. **Seated Forward Fold:** Sit towards the front edge of your chair with your feet hip-width apart. Inhale to lengthen your spine, then exhale as you hinge forward from your hips, reaching towards your feet or the floor. Hold for a few breaths, then slowly return to an upright position.

4. **Ankle Circles:** Sit comfortably in your chair and lift one foot off the floor. Rotate your ankle in a circular motion, first clockwise and then counterclockwise. Repeat on the other side.

5. **Wrist Stretch:** Extend your right arm in front of you with the palm facing down. Use your left hand to gently press down on your right fingertips, stretching the wrist and forearm. Hold for a few breaths, then switch sides.

6. **Shoulder Rolls:** Sit comfortably in your chair with your feet flat on the floor. Inhale as you lift your shoulders up towards your ears, then exhale as you roll them back and down. Repeat several times, moving with your breath.

Tips for Practicing Chair Yoga with Arthritis:

1. **Listen to Your Body:** Pay attention to how your body feels during chair yoga practice and modify poses as needed to avoid discomfort or pain.

2. **Move Mindfully:** Practice gentle, controlled movements, and avoid jerky or sudden motions that could aggravate arthritis symptoms.

3. **Use Props:** Consider using props such as blankets, blocks, or cushions to support your body and make poses more accessible.

4. **Stay Consistent:** Practice chair yoga regularly to experience the full benefits. Even short sessions a few times a week can make a difference in managing arthritis symptoms.

5. **Consult a Professional:** If you have severe arthritis or other health concerns, consult with a healthcare professional before starting a new exercise program, including chair yoga.

Conclusion:

Chair yoga can be a valuable tool for managing arthritis and joint pain, providing gentle movement, relaxation, and stress relief. By incorporating chair yoga into your daily routine, you can improve joint mobility, reduce stiffness, and increase flexibility while promoting overall well-being. With regular practice and mindful awareness, chair yoga can help individuals living with arthritis maintain an active and fulfilling lifestyle, allowing them to move with greater ease and comfort.

6.3 Alleviating Back Pain and Improving Spinal Health with Chair Yoga

Back pain and spinal issues can significantly impact daily life, causing discomfort, limited mobility, and reduced quality of life. Chair yoga offers a gentle and effective approach to alleviating back pain, improving spinal health, and promoting overall well-being. By incorporating mindful movements, gentle stretches, and breath awareness, chair yoga can help relieve tension, increase flexibility, and strengthen the muscles that support the spine. Let's explore how chair yoga can be used to alleviate back pain and improve spinal health:

Understanding Back Pain and Spinal Health:

Back pain can arise from various factors, including poor posture, muscle imbalances, injury, or conditions such as herniated discs or spinal stenosis. Maintaining spinal health is crucial for overall well-being, as the spine provides support, protection, and mobility for the entire body. By addressing muscle imbalances, promoting proper alignment, and increasing flexibility, individuals can experience relief from back pain and improve spinal health.

Benefits of Chair Yoga for Back Pain and Spinal Health:

1. **Gentle Stretching:** Chair yoga includes gentle stretches that target the muscles of the back, hips, and spine, helping to release tension and improve flexibility.

2. **Core Strengthening:** Many chair yoga poses engage the core muscles, which support the spine and help maintain proper posture, reducing the risk of back pain and injury.

"Zen Seats: Chair Yoga Mastery for Vibrant Seniors"

3. **Improved Posture:** Chair yoga promotes awareness of posture and alignment, helping individuals develop better postural habits to prevent strain on the spine and alleviate back pain.

4. **Increased Mobility:** Chair yoga encourages movement in all directions, promoting spinal flexibility and mobility, which can alleviate stiffness and reduce discomfort.

5. **Stress Reduction:** Chair yoga incorporates relaxation techniques such as deep breathing and mindfulness, which can help reduce stress levels and tension in the body, contributing to overall spinal health.

Chair Yoga Poses for Alleviating Back Pain and Improving Spinal Health:

1. **Seated Cat-Cow Stretch:** Sit comfortably in your chair with your feet flat on the floor. Inhale as you arch your back and lift your chest (cow pose), then exhale as you round your spine and tuck your chin to your chest (cat pose). Repeat several times, moving with your breath to massage the spine and release tension.

2. **Seated Forward Fold:** Sit towards the front edge of your chair with your feet hip-width apart. Inhale to lengthen your spine, then exhale as you hinge forward from your hips, reaching towards your feet or the floor. Hold for a few breaths, feeling the stretch in your hamstrings and lower back.

3. **Seated Spinal Twist:** Sit upright in your chair with your feet flat on the floor. Inhale to lengthen your

spine, then exhale as you twist to the right, placing your left hand on the outside of your right knee and your right hand on the back of the chair. Hold for a few breaths, then repeat on the other side.

4. **Seated Side Stretch:** Sit comfortably in your chair with your feet flat on the floor. Inhale to lengthen your spine, then exhale as you reach your right arm overhead and lean to the left, feeling the stretch along the right side of your body. Hold for a few breaths, then repeat on the other side.

5. **Chair Cat-Cow Stretch:** Sit towards the front edge of your chair with your feet flat on the floor and your hands resting on your thighs. Inhale as you arch your back and lift your chest, then exhale as you round your spine and tuck your chin to your chest. Continue flowing between cat and cow poses, synchronizing movement with breath.

Tips for Practicing Chair Yoga Safely and Effectively:

1. **Listen to Your Body:** Pay attention to how your body feels during chair yoga practice and modify poses as needed to avoid discomfort or pain.

2. **Engage Your Core:** Activate the core muscles to support your spine and maintain stability during chair yoga poses.

3. **Breathe Mindfully:** Practice deep, diaphragmatic breathing to oxygenate the body, promote relaxation, and enhance the benefits of chair yoga for back pain and spinal health.

4. **Be Consistent:** Practice chair yoga regularly to experience the full benefits. Even short sessions a few times a week can make a significant difference in alleviating back pain and improving spinal health.

5. **Consult a Professional:** If you have severe back pain or underlying spinal issues, consult with a healthcare professional before starting a new exercise program, including chair yoga.

Conclusion:

Chair yoga offers a gentle and accessible approach to alleviating back pain, improving spinal health, and promoting overall well-being. By incorporating mindful movements, gentle stretches, and breath awareness, individuals can experience relief from back discomfort, increase flexibility, and strengthen the muscles that support the spine. With regular practice and mindful awareness, chair yoga can be a valuable tool for enhancing spinal health and enjoying a life free from back.

6.4 Nurturing Mind, Body, and Spirit: The Holistic Approach to Well-being

In the pursuit of a fulfilling and balanced life, nurturing the mind, body, and spirit is essential. This holistic approach to well-being recognizes the interconnectedness of these aspects of our being and emphasizes the importance of caring for each dimension to achieve optimal health and happiness. Let's explore what it means to nurture the mind, body, and spirit, and how we can cultivate a harmonious balance in our lives:

Understanding Mind, Body, and Spirit:

1. **Mind:** The mind encompasses our thoughts, beliefs, emotions, and mental processes. It governs our perception of the world, our ability to reason and problem-solve, and our capacity for self-awareness and introspection.

2. **Body:** The body refers to our physical form, including our anatomy, physiology, and overall health. It encompasses our physical sensations, movements, and bodily functions, as well as our sensory experiences and interactions with the external environment.

3. **Spirit:** The spirit represents our inner essence or core being, often associated with our sense of purpose, meaning, and connection to something greater than ourselves. It encompasses our values, beliefs, creativity, intuition, and sense of interconnectedness with all living beings.

"Zen Seats: Chair Yoga Mastery for Vibrant Seniors"

The Importance of Holistic Well-being:

Nurturing the mind, body, and spirit is essential for achieving holistic well-being and living a fulfilling life. When one aspect of our being is out of balance, it can impact other areas and contribute to feelings of dis-ease or imbalance. By addressing the needs of the mind, body, and spirit, we can cultivate greater harmony, resilience, and vitality in our lives.

Practices for Nurturing Mind, Body, and Spirit:

1. **Mind:**

    - **Mindfulness Meditation:** Cultivate present-moment awareness through mindfulness meditation, observing thoughts and emotions without judgment.

    - **Journaling:** Explore your thoughts, feelings, and experiences through journaling, allowing for greater self-reflection and insight.

    - **Learning:** Engage in lifelong learning and intellectual pursuits to stimulate the mind and expand your knowledge and understanding of the world.

2. **Body:**

    - **Physical Exercise:** Incorporate regular exercise into your routine, including activities such as yoga, walking, swimming, or dancing to promote physical fitness and vitality.

- **Nutrition:** Nourish your body with wholesome, nutrient-rich foods that support optimal health and vitality, and practice mindful eating to savor and enjoy your meals.
- **Rest and Relaxation:** Prioritize adequate rest and relaxation to rejuvenate your body and mind, including practices such as sleep hygiene, relaxation techniques, and self-care rituals.

3. **Spirit:**
   - **Nature Connection:** Spend time in nature to foster a sense of connection and awe, appreciating the beauty and interconnectedness of all living beings.
   - **Creative Expression:** Engage in creative activities such as art, music, writing, or gardening to nourish your spirit and tap into your innate creativity and expression.
   - **Spiritual Practices:** Explore spiritual practices that resonate with you, such as prayer, meditation, ritual, or sacred ceremony, to nurture your sense of connection to the divine and the sacred within and around you.

Cultivating Balance and Integration:

Achieving balance and integration among the mind, body, and spirit involves consciously attending to each aspect of our being and fostering a sense of wholeness and harmony. This may involve exploring different practices and modalities that resonate with your unique needs and preferences, as well as honoring your intuition and inner wisdom in guiding your journey of self-discovery and growth.

Conclusion:

Nurturing the mind, body, and spirit is essential for achieving holistic well-being and living a fulfilling life. By cultivating awareness, balance, and integration among these aspects of our being, we can experience greater harmony, resilience, and vitality, allowing us to thrive and flourish in all areas of our lives. Whether through mindfulness meditation, physical exercise, creative expression, or spiritual practices, the key is to prioritize self-care and self-discovery, honoring the interconnectedness of mind, body, and spirit in our journey of personal growth and transformation.

CHAPTER SEVEN

7.1 CULTIVATING SELF-COMPASSION AND ACCEPTANCE THROUGH CHAIR YOGA

Chair yoga offers a gentle and accessible way to cultivate self-compassion and acceptance, fostering a deeper connection with ourselves and promoting emotional well-being. By integrating mindful movement, breath awareness, and relaxation techniques, chair yoga provides a supportive space for practicing self-love, kindness, and acceptance. Let's explore how chair yoga can be a powerful tool for cultivating self-compassion and acceptance:

Understanding Self-Compassion and Acceptance:

1. **Self-Compassion:** Self-compassion involves treating ourselves with kindness, understanding, and care, especially in times of struggle, failure, or suffering. It involves acknowledging our humanity, embracing our imperfections, and offering ourselves the same compassion and support we would give to a dear friend.

2. **Acceptance:** Acceptance involves embracing ourselves as we are, without judgment or resistance, and recognizing that all experiences, thoughts, and emotions are valid and worthy of acknowledgment. It involves letting go of the need for perfection or control and embracing the present moment with openness and curiosity.

"Zen Seats: Chair Yoga Mastery for Vibrant Seniors"

Benefits of Chair Yoga for Self-Compassion and Acceptance:

1. **Gentle Movement:** Chair yoga offers gentle movements and stretches that promote relaxation, release tension, and foster a sense of well-being. By moving mindfully and with intention, we can cultivate a deeper connection with our bodies and honor our physical limitations with compassion and acceptance.

2. **Breath Awareness:** Chair yoga emphasizes breath awareness, allowing us to connect with the present moment and cultivate a sense of calmness and presence. By focusing on the breath, we can soothe our nervous system, reduce stress, and cultivate self-compassion and acceptance for our current experience.

3. **Mindfulness:** Chair yoga encourages mindfulness, or present-moment awareness, allowing us to observe our thoughts, feelings, and sensations without judgment. By practicing non-reactivity and self-compassion, we can cultivate greater acceptance of our inner experiences and develop a sense of inner peace and resilience.

4. **Relaxation Techniques:** Chair yoga incorporates relaxation techniques such as guided imagery, progressive muscle relaxation, and deep breathing exercises, which promote relaxation, reduce stress, and foster a sense of well-being. By practicing self-soothing techniques, we can cultivate self-compassion and acceptance for ourselves and our experiences.

"Zen Seats: Chair Yoga Mastery for Vibrant Seniors"

Chair Yoga Practices for Cultivating Self-Compassion and Acceptance:

1. **Loving-Kindness Meditation:** Begin your chair yoga practice with a loving-kindness meditation, offering phrases of kindness, compassion, and acceptance to yourself and others. Repeat phrases such as "May I be happy, may I be healthy, may I be at ease" to cultivate a sense of self-compassion and acceptance.

2. **Gentle Movement Sequences:** Flow through gentle movement sequences that honor your body's needs and limitations, moving with compassion and acceptance for yourself as you are in the present moment. Focus on the sensations in your body and move with gentleness and care.

3. **Breath Awareness:** Practice breath awareness throughout your chair yoga practice, focusing on the sensations of the breath as it moves in and out of your body. Notice any thoughts or emotions that arise without judgment, allowing them to come and go like passing clouds in the sky.

4. **Body Scan Relaxation:** Practice a body scan relaxation exercise, bringing your awareness to each part of your body from head to toe, noticing any areas of tension or discomfort with kindness and acceptance. Use the breath to release tension and promote relaxation throughout your body.

"Zen Seats: Chair Yoga Mastery for Vibrant Seniors"

Tips for Cultivating Self-Compassion and Acceptance through Chair Yoga:

1. **Be Gentle with Yourself:** Approach your chair yoga practice with gentleness and compassion, honoring your body's needs and limitations without judgment or self-criticism.

2. **Practice Non-Judgment:** Cultivate an attitude of non-judgment and acceptance towards your thoughts, feelings, and experiences during chair yoga practice, allowing them to arise and pass without clinging or resistance.

3. **Set Intentions:** Set intentions for your chair yoga practice that reflect self-compassion and acceptance, such as "May I be kind to myself" or "May I accept myself as I am."

4. **Use Affirmations:** Incorporate affirmations or positive statements into your chair yoga practice that affirm your worthiness, such as "I am enough" or "I deserve love and compassion."

5. **Extend Kindness to Others:** Extend the practice of self-compassion and acceptance to others in your life, cultivating kindness, empathy, and understanding towards all beings.

Conclusion:

Chair yoga provides a nurturing space for cultivating self-compassion and acceptance, fostering a deeper connection with ourselves and promoting emotional well-being. By integrating mindful movement, breath awareness, and relaxation techniques into our practice, we can cultivate a sense of kindness, understanding, and acceptance for ourselves and our experiences. Whether through loving-kindness meditation, gentle movement sequences, or breath awareness exercises, chair yoga offers a powerful pathway to self-compassion and acceptance, allowing us to embrace ourselves as we are and cultivate greater peace, resilience, and well-being in our lives.

7.2 Connecting with Others through Chair Yoga Communities and Classes

Chair yoga communities and classes offer a unique opportunity to connect with others, cultivate meaningful relationships, and foster a sense of belonging and support. Whether in-person or online, chair yoga communities provide a supportive environment where individuals can come together to practice yoga, share experiences, and uplift one another. Let's explore how chair yoga communities and classes facilitate connection and enhance well-being:

Creating Community and Connection:

1. **Shared Experience:** Chair yoga communities bring together individuals who share a common interest in yoga and well-being, creating a sense of camaraderie and connection. Practicing yoga together fosters a shared experience that can deepen relationships and build a sense of community.

2. **Supportive Environment:** Chair yoga classes offer a supportive environment where individuals of all ages, abilities, and backgrounds can come together to practice yoga in a safe and inclusive space. Instructors and fellow participants provide

encouragement, guidance, and support, fostering a sense of belonging and acceptance.

3. **Social Interaction:** Chair yoga communities provide opportunities for social interaction and engagement, allowing participants to connect with others, make new friends, and build meaningful relationships. Socializing before or after class, participating in group activities, or attending community events can further strengthen bonds and enhance connection.

Benefits of Connecting through Chair Yoga:

1. **Emotional Support:** Chair yoga communities offer a source of emotional support and companionship, providing a space where individuals can express themselves, share their struggles and triumphs, and receive encouragement and empathy from others.

2. **Sense of Belonging:** Participating in a chair yoga community fosters a sense of belonging and connection, helping individuals feel valued, accepted, and part of something larger than themselves. Belonging to a community can enhance overall well-being and promote a sense of purpose and fulfillment.

3. **Accountability and Motivation:** Being part of a chair yoga community provides accountability and motivation to maintain a regular yoga practice. Connecting with others who share similar goals and interests can inspire individuals to stay committed to their practice and achieve their wellness objectives.

4. **Learning and Growth:** Chair yoga communities offer opportunities for learning and growth,

providing access to experienced instructors, workshops, and educational resources. Engaging with others in the community can expand knowledge, deepen understanding, and inspire personal and spiritual growth.

Ways to Connect with Others through Chair Yoga:

1. **Attend Classes:** Participate in chair yoga classes offered at local yoga studios, community centers, senior centers, or online platforms. Regularly attending classes allows you to connect with fellow participants and build relationships over time.

2. **Join Social Events:** Attend social events, workshops, or retreats organized by chair yoga communities to meet others with similar interests and engage in shared activities outside of class.

3. **Online Communities:** Join online chair yoga communities, forums, or social media groups to connect with like-minded individuals, share experiences, and participate in discussions related to yoga and well-being.

4. **Volunteer or Lead:** Volunteer to assist with chair yoga classes or events, or consider becoming a chair yoga instructor yourself. Taking on leadership roles within the community allows you to connect with others, contribute your skills and expertise, and make a positive impact on the lives of others.

"Zen Seats: Chair Yoga Mastery for Vibrant Seniors"

Cultivating Connection and Well-being:

1. **Openness and Authenticity:** Cultivate openness and authenticity in your interactions with others, allowing yourself to be vulnerable and genuine. Sharing your experiences, challenges, and triumphs fosters deeper connections and promotes a sense of mutual understanding and support.

2. **Active Listening:** Practice active listening and empathy in your interactions with others, showing genuine interest and compassion for their experiences and perspectives. Listening with an open heart and mind fosters meaningful connections and strengthens relationships.

3. **Express Gratitude:** Express gratitude and appreciation for the individuals in your chair yoga community, acknowledging their contributions, kindness, and support. Showing gratitude fosters positivity, strengthens connections, and enhances overall well-being.

Conclusion:

Chair yoga communities and classes provide a valuable opportunity to connect with others, cultivate relationships, and foster a sense of belonging and support. Whether in-person or online, chair yoga communities offer a supportive environment where individuals can come together to practice yoga, share experiences, and uplift one another. By participating in chair yoga classes, attending social events, and engaging with others in the community, individuals can enhance their well-being, cultivate meaningful connections, and experience the transformative power of community support and connection.

7.3 Embracing Aging Gracefully with Chair Yoga Wisdom

Aging is a natural and inevitable part of life, and chair yoga offers a gentle and empowering approach to navigating the aging process with grace, wisdom, and vitality. By embracing the principles of chair yoga, individuals can cultivate resilience, maintain physical and mental well-being, and enhance their overall quality of life as they age. Let's explore how chair yoga wisdom can support individuals in embracing aging gracefully:

Understanding Aging with Grace:

1. **Acceptance:** Embracing aging gracefully begins with acceptance of the natural changes that occur as we grow older. Accepting the passage of time and the changes in our bodies allows us to approach aging with grace and resilience.

2. **Self-Compassion:** Practicing self-compassion involves treating ourselves with kindness, understanding, and acceptance as we navigate the challenges and joys of aging. Cultivating self-compassion allows us to embrace our imperfections and celebrate our inherent worthiness at every stage of life.

3. **Adaptability:** Embracing aging gracefully requires adaptability and flexibility in both body and mind. Being open to change, learning new skills, and adapting to shifting circumstances allows us to navigate the aging process with resilience and vitality.

"Zen Seats: Chair Yoga Mastery for Vibrant Seniors"

Chair Yoga Wisdom for Aging Gracefully:

1. **Gentle Movement:** Chair yoga emphasizes gentle movements and stretches that promote flexibility, mobility, and strength, making it an ideal practice for individuals of all ages and abilities. By incorporating gentle movement into daily life, individuals can maintain physical function and vitality as they age.

2. **Breath Awareness:** Chair yoga emphasizes breath awareness, encouraging individuals to connect with the breath as a source of vitality and presence. Practicing deep, mindful breathing can reduce stress, promote relaxation, and enhance overall well-being, supporting individuals in navigating the challenges of aging with grace and ease.

3. **Mindfulness:** Chair yoga cultivates mindfulness, or present-moment awareness, allowing individuals to fully engage with the present moment and savor the richness of life as it unfolds. By practicing mindfulness, individuals can develop greater resilience, clarity, and appreciation for the beauty and wisdom of aging.

4. **Self-Care:** Chair yoga promotes self-care practices that nurture the body, mind, and spirit, allowing individuals to prioritize their well-being and vitality as they age. Engaging in regular self-care rituals, such as meditation, relaxation techniques, and nourishing movement, supports individuals in maintaining balance and harmony in their lives.

5. **Community Connection:** Chair yoga communities provide a supportive environment where individuals can connect with others, share experiences, and

cultivate meaningful relationships. Building connections with like-minded individuals fosters a sense of belonging and support, enhancing overall well-being and resilience in the face of aging.

Tips for Embracing Aging Gracefully with Chair Yoga Wisdom:

1. **Start Where You Are:** Embrace your current level of ability and meet yourself with compassion and acceptance as you begin your chair yoga practice. Allow yourself to progress at your own pace and celebrate each step forward on your journey of aging gracefully.

2. **Listen to Your Body:** Honor your body's needs and limitations, modifying poses as needed to accommodate any physical challenges or discomfort. Tune into your body's signals and practice self-care by resting when needed and listening to your body's wisdom.

3. **Cultivate Gratitude:** Cultivate gratitude for the gifts and blessings of aging, embracing the wisdom, experience, and opportunities that come with each passing year. Focus on the positives in your life and celebrate the richness and depth that aging brings.

4. **Stay Curious:** Approach the aging process with curiosity and an open mind, exploring new possibilities, interests, and experiences that bring joy and fulfillment. Stay engaged with life, pursuing hobbies, passions, and relationships that nourish your spirit and ignite your sense of wonder.

5. **Seek Support:** Reach out for support from chair yoga instructors, healthcare professionals, and supportive communities as you navigate the challenges of aging. Surround yourself with individuals who uplift and inspire you, and lean on their wisdom, guidance, and encouragement along the way.

Conclusion:

Chair yoga wisdom offers a holistic approach to embracing aging gracefully, supporting individuals in maintaining physical, mental, and emotional well-being as they grow older. By practicing gentle movement, breath awareness, mindfulness, and self-care, individuals can cultivate resilience, vitality, and inner peace in the face of aging. Embracing the principles of chair yoga wisdom allows individuals to navigate the aging process with grace, wisdom, and vitality, embracing each moment with open arms and a heart full of gratitude.

CHAPTER EIGHT
CONCLUSION

As you reach the conclusion of your chair yoga journey, take a moment to reflect on the path you've traveled and the experiences you've encountered along the way. Consider how chair yoga has impacted your life, both physically and emotionally, and reflect on the insights and lessons you've gained throughout your practice. Take stock of the challenges you've faced and the growth you've experienced, recognizing the resilience and strength that have emerged as a result of your dedication to your practice.

Celebrate your progress and achievements in your chair yoga practice, acknowledging the strides you've made and the milestones you've reached. Whether you've improved your flexibility, reduced stress, or deepened your sense of self-awareness, take pride in the progress you've achieved and the positive changes you've experienced. Celebrate the dedication and effort you've invested in your practice, honoring the commitment you've made to your own well-being and personal growth.

As you conclude your chair yoga journey, consider how you can continue to nurture your practice and share the gift of chair yoga with others. Commit to maintaining a regular practice that supports your physical, mental, and emotional well-being, integrating chair yoga into your daily routine as a source of strength, balance, and vitality. Additionally, consider how you can share your knowledge and experience with others, whether by teaching chair yoga classes, leading workshops, or simply introducing friends and loved ones to the benefits of chair yoga. By continuing to cultivate your

"Zen Seats: Chair Yoga Mastery for Vibrant Seniors"

practice and share its benefits with others, you contribute to the well-being and transformation of yourself and those around you.

In conclusion, your chair yoga journey is a testament to your dedication, resilience, and commitment to your own well-being. As you reflect on your journey, celebrate your progress, and continue your practice, may you find joy, fulfillment, and inner peace on the path ahead.

THANKS FOR READING

"Zen Seats: Chair Yoga Mastery for Vibrant Seniors"

www.ingramcontent.com/pod-product-compliance
Lightning Source LLC
Chambersburg PA
CBHW071058240526
45471CB00016B/2149